LUPUS DIET COOKBOOK FOR BEGINNERS

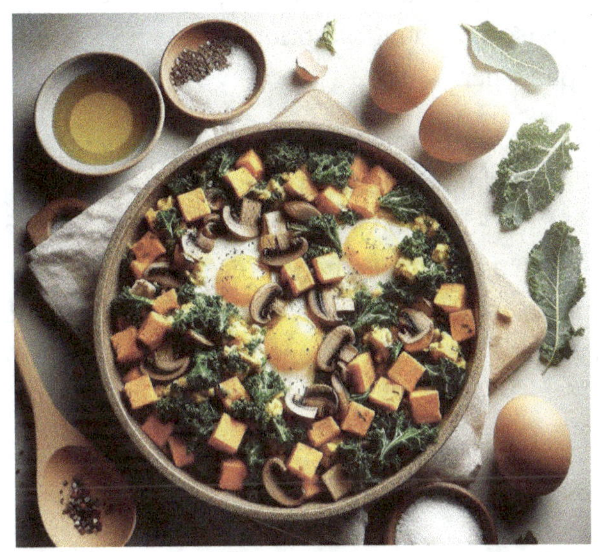

Delicious Anti-Lupus Recipes and Diet Plan to Soothe Inflammation and Live Healthier

Robert Elliot

Copyright © Robert Elliot (2024)

The contents of this book are based on the author's research, knowledge, and experience. They are meant for educational purposes only and should not be taken as medical advice. Readers should consult their healthcare provider before making any changes to their health regimen.

Table of Contents

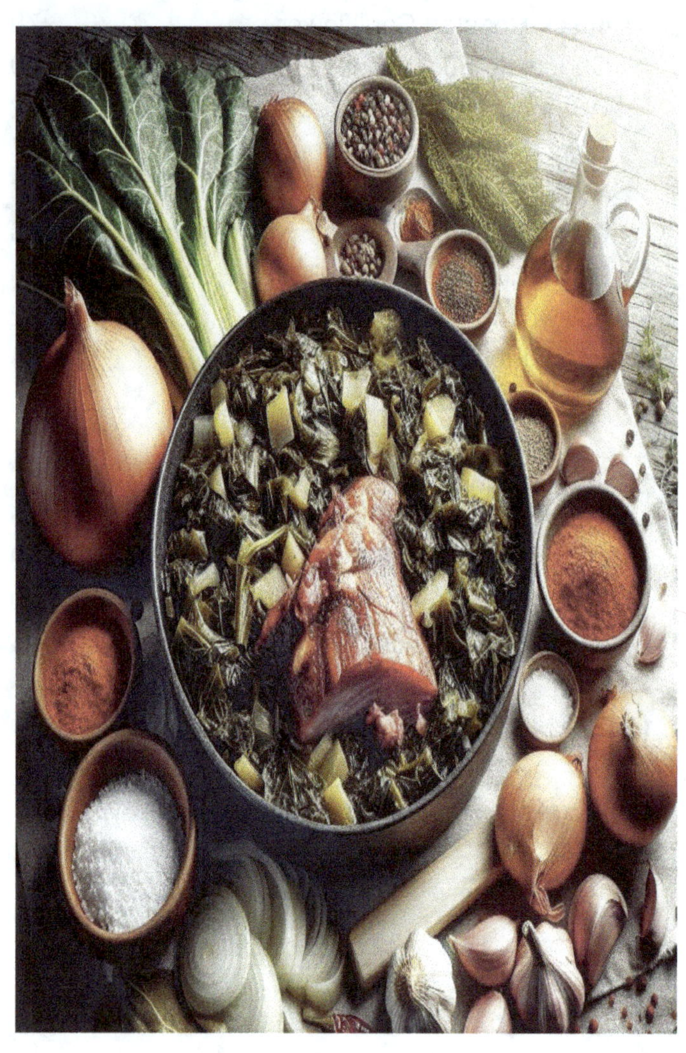

Introduction

When my aunty, Aunt Marie, started having lupus-like symptoms, it felt like a rogue Uber driver had hijacked her life. One minute she was salsa-ing at weddings, the next she was battling fatigue that could floor a heavyweight. Her vibrant laugh, once as infectious as a TikTok dance craze, became a whisper. The woman who'd taught me to fold dumplings with flour-dusted fingers was now struggling to hold a spoon.

I'm a doctor and nutritionist who's seen my fair share of medical battles. But lupus? It was a beast I hadn't tamed. It stole Marie's energy, her appetite, her freaking joy. Watching her shrink, her cheekbones sharpening like winter knives, was like watching a favorite song fade to static.

Except, that's not the end of the story. Because Marie, bless her stubborn soul, refused to be a passive passenger in this Uber ride from hell. She started researching, sniffing out every morsel of information about lupus like a truffle pig on a mission. And guess what? She found a secret weapon: food.

Not kale smoothies and chia pudding, mind you. This was a delicious rebellion, a fiesta of flavors that fought back against the inflammation. Spicy salmon with roasted veggies, sunshine-yellow turmeric lattes, and blueberry-packed muffins that tasted like defiance. Marie's kitchen became an alchemist's lab, each dish a potion brewed to reclaim her health.

And it worked. Slowly, like a sunrise chasing away the night, Marie's color returned. Her laugh, once a ghost, filled the room again. She still had flare-ups, sure, but now she had a toolbox – a pantry full of ammunition, a fridge stocked with sunshine.

This book, my friends, is that toolbox. It's the map Aunt Marie drew, the battle plan she forged in her kitchen. It's for everyone who's ever felt like lupus is driving their life, for anyone who wants to reclaim their health, one delicious bite at a time. So, grab your apron, crank up the music, and let's cook our way back to badass. You ready? Let's go.

Chapter 1:
Understanding Lupus and Nutrition

What is Lupus?

Lupus is a long-term autoimmune condition that affects various parts of the body. The immune system, which normally protects against viruses, bacteria, and other foreign invaders, becomes hyperactive and attacks healthy tissues. This can lead to inflammation, pain, and damage to joints, skin, kidneys, heart, lungs, brain, and blood cells.

Common Symptoms:
- Fatigue
- Joint pain and swelling
- Skin rashes, often exacerbated by sun exposure
- Fever
- Kidney problems
- Chest pain during deep breaths
- Unexplained hair loss

Understanding the nature of lupus is crucial for individuals navigating its challenges. While there is no cure, proper management strategies, including dietary choices, can significantly impact the quality of life for those with lupus.

The Connection Between Lupus and Diet

The Immune System and Inflammation:
In lupus, the immune system mistakenly identifies healthy tissues as threats, leading to chronic inflammation. This inflammation is a key player in lupus symptoms. Nutrition plays a pivotal role in managing inflammation, and certain foods can either exacerbate or alleviate these symptoms.

Lupus Triggers and Food Sensitivities:
Understanding potential triggers is essential. Some individuals with lupus may experience increased symptoms with certain foods, while others may find relief by incorporating anti-inflammatory options into their diet.

The Importance of a Balanced Diet:
Maintaining a well-balanced diet is crucial for overall health, especially for those with lupus. Key components include:
- **Essential Vitamins**: A, C, D, and E.
- **Omega-3 Fatty Acids**: Found in fatty fish, flaxseeds, and walnuts.
- **Antioxidants**: Present in colorful fruits and vegetables, helping to combat oxidative stress.

Avoiding Lupus Flare Triggers:
Certain foods may trigger lupus flares or exacerbate symptoms. These can include excessive alcohol, processed foods, and those high in saturated fats. Identifying and avoiding these triggers is a crucial aspect of managing lupus through nutrition.

Collaboration with Healthcare Professionals:
Before making significant dietary changes, individuals with lupus should consult with healthcare professionals, including rheumatologists and nutritionists. A personalized approach ensures that dietary adjustments align with overall treatment plans and individual health needs.

The Holistic Approach:
This cookbook embraces a holistic approach to lupus management. By understanding the connection between lupus and nutrition, individuals can make informed choices to enhance their well-being. This cookbook is not just about what to eat but about fostering a positive relationship with food, empowering readers to make choices that contribute to a healthier, more balanced life.

Understanding lupus and its connection to nutrition sets the stage for the recipes and insights that follow. Let's embark on this journey toward better health together.

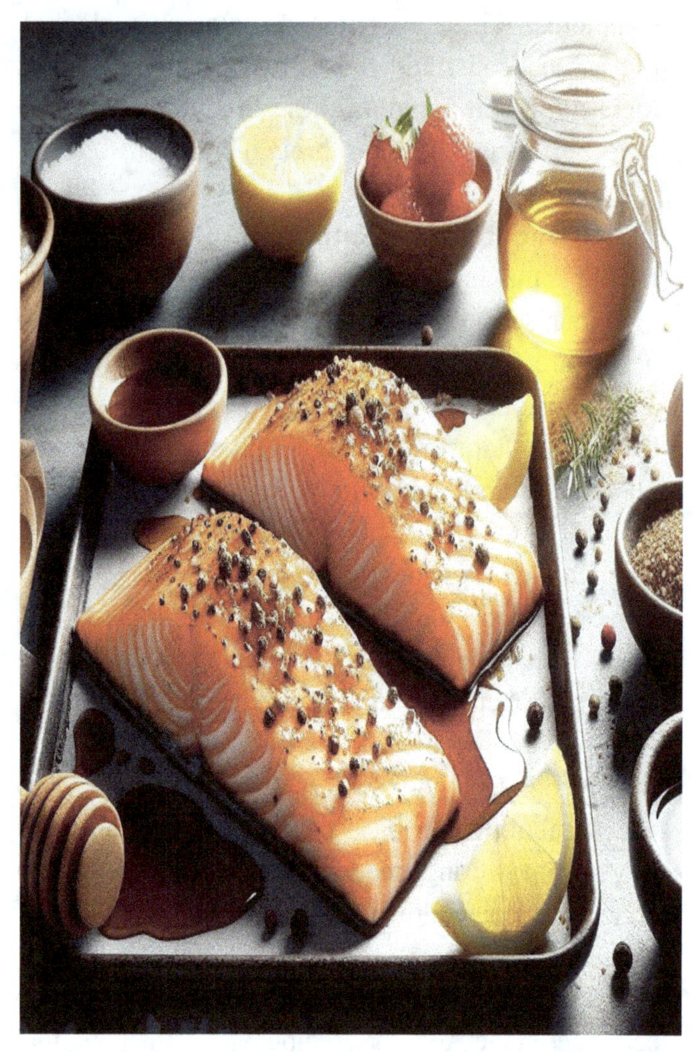

Chapter 2: Building a Lupus-Friendly Plate

Anti-Inflammatory Foods

In the realm of lupus management, the importance of incorporating anti-inflammatory foods into your diet cannot be overstated. These foods have the power to mitigate inflammation, a key factor in lupus symptoms.

- **Leafy Greens**:Packed with vitamins A, C, and K, leafy greens like kale, spinach, and Swiss chard provide a nutrient-rich foundation for lupus-friendly meals.

- **Berries**: Loaded with antioxidants, berries such as blueberries, strawberries, and raspberries contribute not only to a flavorful diet but also help combat oxidative stress.

- **Fatty Fish**: The fish species salmon, mackerel, and sardines are high in omega-3 fatty acids. These healthy fats have anti-inflammatory properties, promoting joint health and overall well-being.

- **Turmeric**: Known for its active compound curcumin, turmeric possesses potent anti-inflammatory and antioxidant effects. Including this spice in your meals can be a flavorful way to reduce inflammation.

- **Nuts and Seeds**: Almonds, walnuts, flaxseeds, and chia seeds are excellent sources of omega-3s and other nutrients. They make for convenient snacks or additions to salads and smoothies.

Nutrient-Rich Choices

- **Colorful Fruits**: Incorporating a variety of colorful fruits ensures a diverse range of vitamins and antioxidants. Oranges, papayas, and mangoes are rich in vitamin C, vital for immune health.

- **Lean Proteins**: Chicken, turkey, tofu, and legumes offer lean protein sources without the saturated fats found in some red meats. Protein is essential for muscle health and overall energy.

- **Whole Grains**: Choose whole grains such as oats, quinoa, and brown rice. These grains provide complex carbohydrates and fiber, promoting digestive health and stable energy levels.

- **Dairy or Dairy Alternatives**: Calcium is crucial for bone health, especially for individuals with lupus who may be prone to osteoporosis. Incorporate low-fat dairy or fortified dairy alternatives into your diet.

- **Healthy Oils**: Use heart-healthy oils like olive oil, which contains monounsaturated fats and has anti-inflammatory properties. These oils can be the basis for lupus-friendly dressings and cooking.

Practical Tips for Building Your Plate

1. Prioritize Variety:
Aim for a colorful plate, as different colors often signify different nutrients. Variety guarantees that you get a wide range of minerals and vitamins..

2. Portion Control:
Maintain balance by being mindful of portion sizes. This helps prevent overeating and supports overall health.

3. Hydration Matters:

Water is essential for everyone, but especially for those with lupus. Stay hydrated to support kidney function and overall well-being.

4. Read Labels:

Be aware of hidden sugars, excessive sodium, and processed additives. Whenever possible, choose whole, minimally processed meals.

5. Experiment with Flavors:

Spices such as ginger, garlic, and cinnamon can add depth to your dishes without relying on excessive salt or sugar.

By building a lupus-friendly plate with a focus on anti-inflammatory foods and nutrient-rich choices, you lay the foundation for a balanced and supportive diet. Let's now explore how these principles can be applied to create delicious and nourishing meals in the recipes that follow.

Chapter 3: Dietary Restrictions and Considerations

Living with Lupus often means navigating a maze of information and conflicting advice when it comes to food. While a Lupus-friendly diet focuses on anti-inflammatory foods and essential nutrients, there are additional factors to consider, like potential triggers, sensitivities, and restrictions. This chapter is your guide through this maze, empowering you to make informed choices about what works best for your body.

The Trigger Maze: Identifying Your Individual Food Sensitivities

Some individuals with Lupus experience symptoms like joint pain, fatigue, or skin rashes after consuming certain foods. These "trigger foods" vary from person to person, making it crucial to identify yours through a process of observation and elimination. Here are some potential culprits:

- **Gluten**: For some, gluten-containing grains like wheat, barley, and rye can exacerbate symptoms. Consider a trial period of a gluten-free diet to see if it makes a difference.

- **Solanaceous vegetables**: Nightshades like tomatoes, peppers, potatoes, and eggplant have been linked to Lupus flares in some studies. Experiment with eliminating these and reintroducing them to see if they trigger symptoms.
- **Processed foods**: High in sugar, saturated fat, and sodium, processed foods can contribute to inflammation and worsen Lupus symptoms. Choose whole, unprocessed meals whenever you can.
- **Dairy**: Lactose intolerance or sensitivity to dairy protein can cause digestive issues and potentially worsen Lupus symptoms. Explore dairy-free alternatives like lactose-free milk or plant-based cheeses.

Restriction Crossroads: Adapting Your Diet to Suit Your Needs

Beyond potential triggers, other factors might necessitate adapting your diet:

- **Medications**: Certain medications interact with specific foods, requiring dietary adjustments. If you have any concerns, always get in touch with your doctor.

- **Kidney involvement**: If Lupus affects your kidneys, limiting sodium and protein intake might be necessary. Your doctor or a registered dietitian will advise you on specific recommendations.

- **Weight management**: Maintaining a healthy weight is crucial for Lupus management. Your doctor or a dietitian can help you develop a personalized plan for balanced weight management.

Taking a Personalized Approach

Remember, there's no one-size-fits-all Lupus diet. What works for one person might not work for another. The key is to listen to your body, experiment with different approaches, and work closely with your healthcare team to develop a personalized plan that addresses your specific needs and preferences.

Here are some tips for a personalized approach:

- **Keep a food diary**: Track your meals and symptoms to identify potential triggers and patterns.

- **Work with a registered dietitian**: They can assess your individual needs and provide personalized dietary guidance.
- **Join a support group**: Connecting with others facing similar challenges can offer valuable insights and support.
- **Don't be afraid to experiment**: Try new recipes, incorporate different food groups, and find what works best for you.

Remember, navigating the dietary maze with Lupus is about empowerment, not restrictions. By understanding your body's signals, seeking expert advice, and embracing a personalized approach, you can take control of your food choices and build a diet that supports your health and well-being. With each informed bite, you pave the path towards a healthier, happier you, even with Lupus.

Chapter 4: Breakfast

Coconut Banana Breakfast Cookies

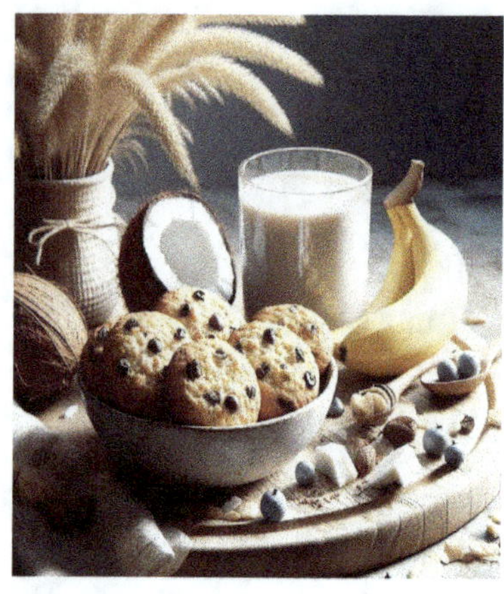

Preparation Time: 15 minutes
Cooking Time: 15 minutes
Servings: 12 cookies

Ingredients:
- 2 ripe bananas, mashed
- 1 ½ cups rolled oats
- 1 cup shredded coconut
- ½ cup almond butter
- ¼ cup maple syrup
- 1 teaspoon vanilla extract
- 1 teaspoon baking powder
- ¼ teaspoon salt

Directions:
1. Preheat oven to 350°F (175°C).

2. In a bowl, mix mashed bananas, rolled oats, shredded coconut, almond butter, maple syrup, vanilla extract, baking powder, and salt.
3. Form cookies on a baking sheet and bake for 15 minutes.

Nutritional Values (per serving):
Calories: 150 | Fat: 7g | Cholesterol: 0mg |
Carbs: 20g | Fiber: 3g | Protein: 3g |
Sodium: 50mg

Coconut Pudding

Preparation Time: 10 minutes
Cooking Time: 15 minutes (plus chilling)
Servings: 4

Ingredients:
- 2 cups coconut milk
- ½ cup sugar
- 3 tablespoons cornstarch
- 1 teaspoon vanilla extract

Directions:
1. In a saucepan, whisk together coconut milk, sugar, cornstarch, and vanilla extract.
2. Cook over medium heat until thickened. Chill before serving.

Nutritional Values (per serving):
Calories: 200 | Fat: 15g | Cholesterol: 0mg |
Carbs: 15g | Fiber: 1g | Protein: 1g |
Sodium: 20mg

Chia Seed Pudding

Preparation Time: 5 minutes (plus chilling)
Cooking Time: 0 minutes
Servings: 2

Ingredients:
- ½ cup chia seeds
- 2 cups almond milk
- 2 tablespoons honey
- 1 teaspoon vanilla extract

Directions:
1. In a bowl, mix chia seeds, almond milk, honey, and vanilla extract.
2. Refrigerate until a pudding-like consistency is reached.

Nutritional Values (per serving):
Calories: 180 | Fat: 10g | Cholesterol: 0mg |
Carbs: 20g | Fiber: 10g | Protein: 4g |
Sodium: 30mg

Chocolate Banana Smoothie

Prep Time: 5 minutes | Cooking Time: 0 minutes | Servings: 2

Ingredients:
- 2 ripe bananas
- 1 cup milk (any type)
- 2 tablespoons cocoa powder
- 1 tablespoon honey
- 1/2 cup ice cubes

Directions:
1. Peel and slice the ripe bananas.
2. In a blender, combine sliced bananas, milk, cocoa powder, honey, and ice cubes.
3. Blend on high speed until the mixture is smooth and creamy.
4. Serve the smoothie right away after pouring it into glasses.

Nutritional Values (per serving):
Calories: 150 | Fat: 2g | Cholesterol: 5mg |
Carbs: 35g | Fiber: 5g | Protein: 3g |
Sodium: 30mg

Breakfast Burrito Bowl

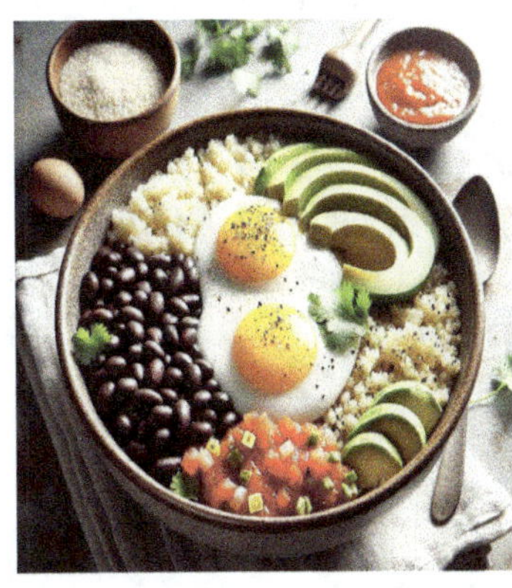

Preparation Time: 15 minutes
Cooking Time: 10 minutes
Servings: 2

Ingredients:
- 1 cup cooked quinoa
- 1/2 cup black beans (canned, drained)
- 1 avocado (sliced)
- 2 eggs (fried)
- Salsa
- Cilantro (optional)

Directions:
1. Cook quinoa according to package instructions.
2. In bowls, layer cooked quinoa, black beans, sliced avocado, and fried eggs.
3. Top with salsa and sprinkle with cilantro if desired.

4. Mix the ingredients in the bowl thoroughly before serving.

Nutritional Values (per serving):
Calories: 450 | Fat: 22g | Cholesterol: 185mg |
Carbs: 45g | Fiber: 12g | Protein: 20g |
Sodium: 320mg

Cauliflower Hash Browns

Prep Time: 15 minutes | Cooking Time: 15 minutes | Servings: 4

Ingredients:
- 1 head cauliflower (grated)
- 2 eggs
- 1/2 cup almond flour
- 1/4 cup grated Parmesan cheese
- 1 teaspoon garlic powder
- Salt and pepper to taste

Directions:
1. Grate the cauliflower using a box grater.
2. In a large bowl, mix grated cauliflower, eggs, almond flour, grated Parmesan cheese, garlic powder, salt, and pepper.
3. Form the mixture into patties.
4. Cook the patties on a skillet over medium heat until both sides are golden brown.

Nutritional Values (per serving):
Calories: 120 | Fat: 7g | Cholesterol: 95mg | Carbs: 10g | Fiber: 4g | Protein: 8g | Sodium: 160mg

---

Hearty Blueberry Pancakes

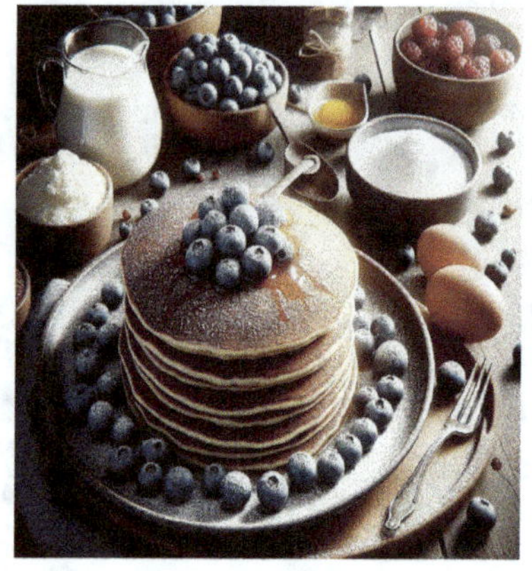

Preparation Time: 10 minutes
Cooking Time: 15 minutes
Servings: 2

Ingredients:
- 1 cup whole wheat flour
- 1 tablespoon sugar
- 1 teaspoon baking powder
- 1/2 teaspoon baking soda
- 1/4 teaspoon salt
- 1 cup buttermilk
- 1 egg
- 1 tablespoon melted butter
- 1/2 cup blueberries

Directions:

1. In a large bowl, whisk together whole wheat flour, sugar, baking powder, baking soda, and salt.

2. In another bowl, whisk together buttermilk, egg, and melted butter. Mix the wet and dry ingredients together until they are well blended.

3. Gently fold in blueberries.

4. Heat a griddle or skillet over medium heat and cook spoonfuls of batter until bubbles form on the surface, then flip and cook until the other side is golden brown.

Nutritional Values (per serving):
Calories: 380 | Fat: 12g | Cholesterol: 105mg |
Carbs: 60g | Fiber: 8g | Protein: 12g |
Sodium: 650mg

Grain-Free Pumpkin Pancakes

Prep Time: 10 minutes | Cooking Time: 10 minutes | Servings: 2

Ingredients:
- 1/2 cup pumpkin puree
- 2 eggs
- 2 tablespoons almond flour
- 1/2 teaspoon baking powder
- 1/2 teaspoon pumpkin spice
- 1/4 teaspoon vanilla extract

Directions:

1. In a bowl, whisk together pumpkin puree, eggs, almond flour, baking powder, pumpkin spice, and vanilla extract until smooth.
2. Over medium heat, preheat a pan or griddle.
3. Spoon the batter onto the griddle to form pancakes and cook until the edges are set, then flip and cook until the other side is golden brown.

Nutritional Values (per serving):
Calories: 210 | Fat: 14g | Cholesterol: 190mg | Carbs: 13g | Fiber: 4g | Protein: 9g | Sodium: 170mg

---

Butternut Squash Porridge

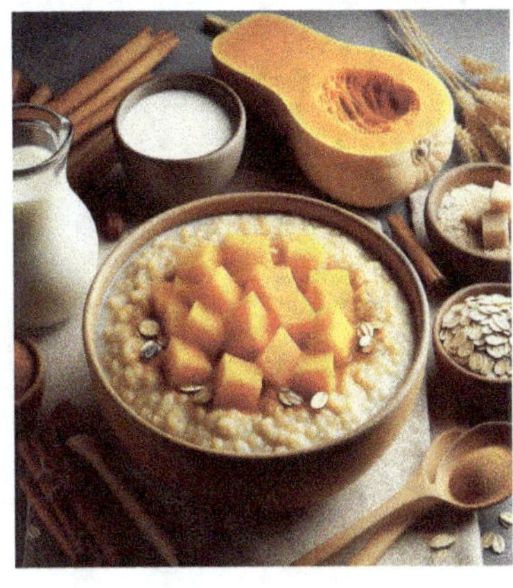

Preparation Time: 15 minutes
Cooking Time: 20 minutes
Servings: 4

Ingredients:
- 2 cups butternut squash (cubed)
- 1 cup steel-cut oats
- 4 cups water
- 1/2 cup milk (any type)
- 2 tablespoons maple syrup
- 1/2 teaspoon cinnamon
- Pinch of salt

Directions:

1. In a large pot, combine butternut squash, steel-cut oats, water, milk, maple syrup, cinnamon, and a pinch of salt.

2. Heat the mixture on medium-high and bring it to a boil.

3. Reduce the heat to low and simmer, stirring occasionally, until the butternut squash is tender and the oats are cooked through.

4. Serve warm.

Nutritional Values (per serving):
Calories: 180 | Fat: 2g | Cholesterol: 2mg |
Carbs: 40g | Fiber: 7g | Protein: 5g |
Sodium: 60mg

Sweet Potato, Kale, and Mushroom Scramble

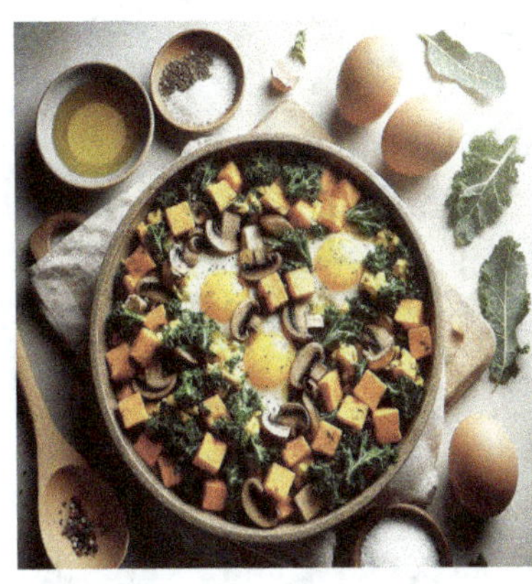

Preparation Time: 15 minutes

Cooking Time: 15 minutes

Servings: 2

Ingredients:
- 1 sweet potato (cubed)
- 1 cup kale (chopped)
-1 cup mushrooms (sliced)
- 4 eggs
- Salt and pepper to taste
- Olive oil for cooking

Directions:
1. Heat olive oil in a large skillet over medium heat.
2. Add the sweet potato cubes and sauté until slightly tender.

3. Stir in the sliced mushrooms and chopped kale, and continue to sauté until the vegetables are cooked through.

4. In a separate bowl, whisk the eggs and season with salt and pepper to taste.

5. Push the vegetables to one side of the skillet and pour the whisked eggs into the empty space.

6. Allow the eggs to set slightly on the bottom, then gently scramble them, incorporating the cooked vegetables.

7. Continue to cook, stirring occasionally, until the eggs are fully cooked and the sweet potatoes are tender.

8. Adjust seasoning if necessary and serve the scramble hot.

Nutritional Values (per serving):
Calories: 320 | Fat: 18g | Cholesterol: 380mg |
Carbs: 28g | Fiber: 5g | Protein: 15g |
Sodium: 260mg

Chapter 5: Lunch

Balsamic Vinaigrette

Ingredients:
- 1/2 cup balsamic vinegar
- 1/4 cup olive oil
- 1 tablespoon Dijon mustard
- 1 clove garlic (minced)
- Salt and pepper to taste

Directions:
1. In a small bowl, whisk together balsamic vinegar, olive oil, Dijon mustard, and minced garlic.
2. Season with salt and pepper to taste.
3. Whisk until well combined.
4. Use immediately or store in a sealed container in the refrigerator.

Nutritional Values (per serving):
Calories: 90 | Fat: 8g | Cholesterol: 0mg |
Carbs: 4g | Fiber: 0g | Protein: 0g |
Sodium: 80mg

Veggie Burrito Bowl

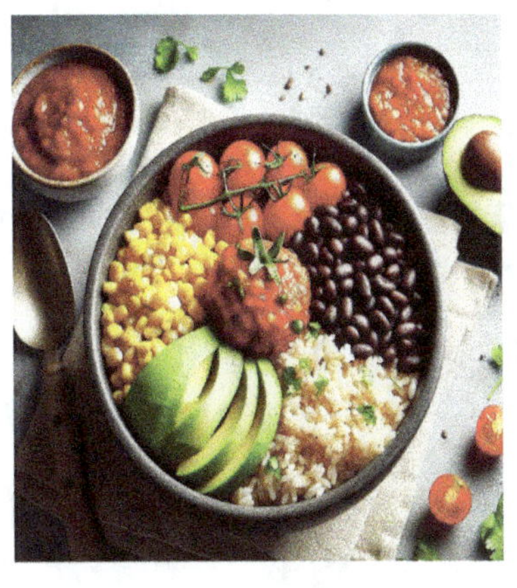

Preparation Time: 15 minutes

Cooking Time: 10 minutes

Servings: 2

Ingredients:
- 1 cup cooked brown rice
- 1 cup black beans (canned, drained)
- 1 cup corn (frozen or canned)
- 1 cup cherry tomatoes (halved)
- 1 avocado (sliced)
- 1/2 cup salsa
- 1/4 cup cilantro (chopped)

Directions:

1. Cook brown rice according to package instructions.

2. In bowls, arrange cooked brown rice, black beans, corn, cherry tomatoes, and sliced avocado.

3. Top with salsa and sprinkle with chopped cilantro.
4. Mix well before enjoying.

Easy Avocado Egg Salad

Prep Time: 10 minutes | Cooking Time: 10 minutes | Servings: 4

Ingredients:
- 4 hard-boiled eggs (chopped)
- 2 ripe avocados (mashed)
- 2 tablespoons Greek yogurt
- 1 tablespoon lemon juice
- Salt and pepper to taste, chives (optional)

Directions:
1. In a bowl, combine chopped hard-boiled eggs, mashed avocados, Greek yogurt, and lemon juice.
2. Mix until well combined.
3. Add pepper and salt to suit your taste.
4. Garnish with chives if desired.
5. Serve as a sandwich filling or on a bed of greens.

Nutritional Values (per serving):
Calories: 220 | Fat: 17g | Cholesterol: 190mg |
Carbs: 9g | Fiber: 6g | Protein: 8g |
Sodium: 120mg

Turmeric Coconut Salmon

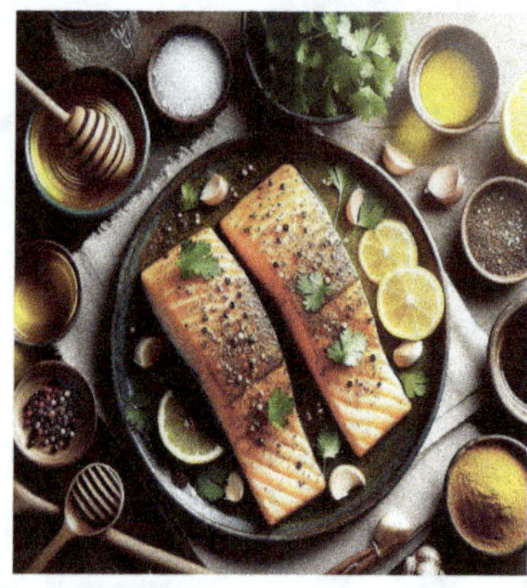

Preparation Time: 15 minutes
Cooking Time: 15 minutes
Servings: 2

Ingredients:
- 2 salmon fillets
- 1 tablespoon turmeric powder
- 1/2 cup coconut milk
- 1 tablespoon soy sauce
- 1 tablespoon honey
- 1 teaspoon minced ginger
- 2 cloves garlic (minced)
- Salt and pepper to taste
- Fresh cilantro for garnish

Directions:
1. Preheat the oven to 375°F (190°C).
2. Arrange the filets of salmon onto a baking sheet.

3. In a bowl, mix turmeric powder, coconut milk, soy sauce, honey, minced ginger, minced garlic, salt, and pepper.
4. Drizzle the mixture onto the salmon filets.
5. Bake for 15 minutes or until the salmon is cooked through.
6. Garnish with fresh cilantro before serving.

Nutritional Values (per serving):
Calories: 350 | Fat: 21g | Cholesterol: 75mg | Carbs: 12g | Fiber: 1g | Protein: 28g | Sodium: 500mg

---

Cucumber Sandwiches

Prep Time: 10 minutes | Cooking Time: 0 minutes | Servings: 4

Ingredients:
- 8 slices whole wheat bread
- 1 cucumber (thinly sliced)
- 1/2 cup cream cheese
- 2 tablespoons fresh dill (chopped)
- Salt and pepper to taste

Directions:
1. Spread cream cheese evenly on each slice of whole wheat bread.
2. Arrange thinly sliced cucumbers on half of the bread slices.
3. Sprinkle chopped fresh dill, salt, and pepper over the cucumbers.
4. Top with the remaining slices of bread to create sandwiches.
5. Cut each sandwich into halves or quarters before serving.

Nutritional Values (per serving):
Calories: 210 | Fat: 9g | Cholesterol: 25mg | Carbs: 28g | Fiber: 5g | Protein: 7g | Sodium: 350mg

---

Bean and Rice Salad

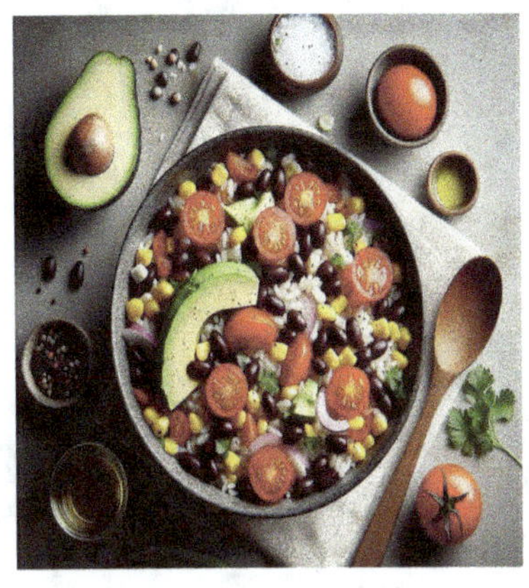

Preparation Time: 15 minutes
Cooking Time: 15 minutes
Servings: 4

Ingredients:
- 1 cup cooked brown rice
- 1 can washed and drained black beans
- 1 cup corn (frozen or canned)
- 1 cup cherry tomatoes (halved)
- 1/2 red onion (finely chopped)
- 1/4 cup fresh cilantro (chopped)
- 1 avocado (diced)
- 2 tablespoons olive oil
- 2 tablespoons lime juice
- Salt and pepper to taste

Directions:
1. In a large bowl, combine cooked brown rice, black beans, corn, cherry tomatoes, red onion, cilantro, and diced avocado.
2. In a small bowl, whisk together olive oil and lime juice.
3. Pour the dressing over the salad and toss until well combined.
4. Season with salt and pepper to taste.
5. Serve chilled.

Nutritional Values (per serving):
Calories: 380 | Fat: 18g | Cholesterol: 0mg |
Carbs: 50g | Fiber: 12g | Protein: 10g |
Sodium: 200mg

Italian Poached Sea Bass

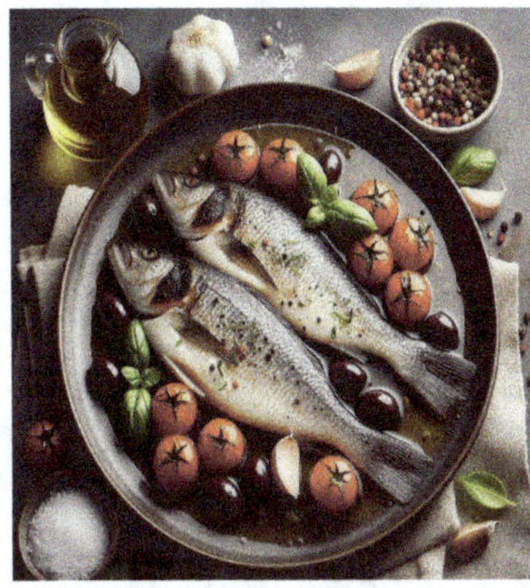

Preparation Time: 10 minutes
Cooking Time: 15 minutes
Servings: 2

Ingredients:
- 2 sea bass fillets
- 1 cup cherry tomatoes (halved)
- 1/2 cup Kalamata olives (pitted and sliced)
- 3 cloves garlic (minced)
- 1/4 cup fresh basil (chopped)
- 2 tablespoons olive oil
- 1/4 cup white wine
- Salt and pepper to taste

Directions:
1. Preheat the oven to 375°F (190°C).
2. Use salt and pepper to season sea bass fillets.

3. In a baking dish, combine cherry tomatoes, Kalamata olives, minced garlic, chopped fresh basil, olive oil, and white wine.

4. Place sea bass fillets on top of the vegetable mixture.

5. Bake for 15 minutes or until the fish is cooked through.

6. Serve the sea bass over the vegetable mixture.

Nutritional Values (per serving):
Calories: 420 | Fat: 23g | Cholesterol: 60mg | Carbs: 10g | Fiber: 3g | Protein: 35g | Sodium: 580mg

---

Slow Cooker Carnitas

Preparation Time: 15 minutes
Cooking Time: 6 hours (slow cooker)
Servings: 8

Ingredients:
- 3 lbs pork shoulder (trimmed and cut into chunks)
- 1 onion (chopped)
- 4 cloves garlic (minced)
- 1 teaspoon cumin
- 1 teaspoon oregano
- 1 teaspoon chili powder
- 1/2 teaspoon smoked paprika
- 1/2 teaspoon salt
- 1/4 teaspoon black pepper
- 1 orange (juiced)
- 1 lime (juiced)

Directions:
1. In a slow cooker, combine pork chunks, chopped onion, minced garlic, cumin, oregano, chili powder, smoked paprika, salt, and black pepper.
2. Squeeze the juice of one orange and one lime over the mixture.

3. Cook on low for 6 hours or until the pork is tender and easily shredded.
4. Preheat the oven to 400°F (200°C).
5. Transfer the shredded pork to a baking sheet and roast for 15 minutes or until edges are crispy.
6. Serve the carnitas in tacos or over rice.

Nutritional Values (per serving):
**Calories: 380 | Fat: 23g | Cholesterol: 110mg |
Carbs: 5g | Fiber: 1g | Protein: 38g |
Sodium: 400mg**

Butternut Squash Soup

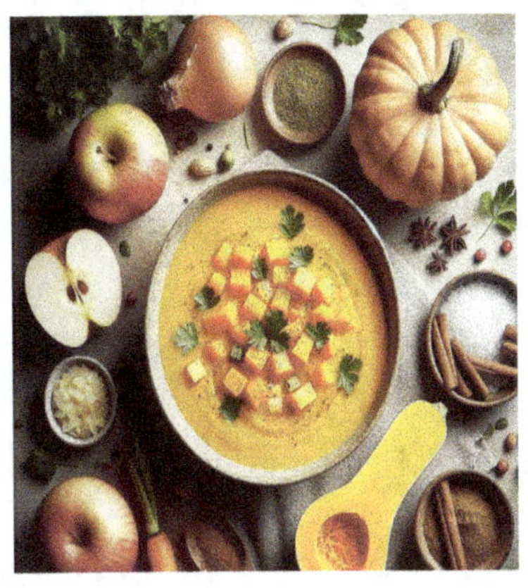

Preparation Time: 15 minutes
Cooking Time: 30 minutes
Servings: 6

Ingredients:
- 1 butternut squash (peeled, seeded, and diced)
- 1 onion (chopped)
- 2 carrots (chopped)
- 2 apples (peeled, cored, and chopped)
- 4 cups vegetable broth
- 1 teaspoon curry powder
- 1/2 teaspoon ground nutmeg
- 1/2 teaspoon cinnamon
- Salt and pepper to taste
- 1/2 cup coconut milk (optional)
- Fresh parsley for garnish

Directions:

1. In a large pot, combine butternut squash, chopped onion, chopped carrots, chopped apples, vegetable broth, curry powder, ground nutmeg, cinnamon, salt, and pepper.

2. Bring to a boil, then reduce heat and simmer for 25-30 minutes or until vegetables are tender.

3. Puree the soup until it's smooth using an immersion blender.

4. Stir in coconut milk if desired.

5. Garnish with fresh parsley before serving.

Nutritional Values (per serving):
Calories: 180 | Fat: 3g | Cholesterol: 0mg |
Carbs: 40g | Fiber: 7g | Protein: 2g |
Sodium: 550mg

Vegetable Stir-Fry

Preparation Time: 15 minutes
Cooking Time: 10 minutes
Servings: 4

Ingredients:
- 2 tablespoons soy sauce
- 1 tablespoon hoisin sauce
- 1 tablespoon sesame oil
- 1 tablespoon vegetable oil
- 2 cloves garlic (minced)
- 1 tablespoon ginger (minced)
- 1 broccoli head (cut into florets)
- 1 bell pepper (sliced)
- 1 carrot (julienned)
- 1 zucchini (sliced)
- 1 cup snap peas
- 1 cup mushrooms (sliced)
- 2 green onions (sliced)
- Sesame seeds for garnish

Directions:
1. Mix the sesame oil, hoisin sauce, and soy sauce in a small bowl.

2. In a wok or large skillet, heat the vegetable oil over high heat.

3. Stir-fry the ginger and minced garlic for 30 seconds.

4. Add broccoli, bell pepper, carrot, zucchini, snap peas, and mushrooms. Stir-fry for 5-7 minutes or until vegetables are crisp-tender.

5. Pour the sauce over the vegetables and toss to coat.

6. Stir in sliced green onions.

7. Garnish with sesame seeds before serving.

Nutritional Values (per serving):
**Calories: 180 | Fat: 9g | Cholesterol: 0mg |
Carbs: 22g | Fiber: 7g | Protein: 10g |
Sodium: 2g**

Chapter 6: Dinner

Mushroom Stroganoff over Mashed Cauliflower

Preparation Time: 15 minutes
Cooking Time: 20 minutes
Servings: 4

Ingredients:
For the Stroganoff:
- 2 cups mushrooms (sliced)
- 1 onion (finely chopped)
- 2 cloves garlic (minced)
- 1 tablespoon olive oil
- 2 tablespoons flour
- 1 cup vegetable broth
- 1 tablespoon soy sauce
- 1 teaspoon Dijon mustard
- Salt and pepper to taste
- Fresh parsley for garnish

For the Mashed Cauliflower:
- 1 head cauliflower (cut into florets)
- 2 tablespoons butter
- 1/4 cup milk (any type)
- Salt and pepper to taste

Directions:

1. In a large skillet, sauté mushrooms, chopped onion, and minced garlic in olive oil until softened.

2. Sprinkle flour over the mushroom mixture, stirring to coat.

3. Gradually add vegetable broth, soy sauce, and Dijon mustard. Stir until the sauce thickens.

4. Season with salt and pepper to taste. Garnish with fresh parsley.

5. For the mashed cauliflower, steam cauliflower florets until tender. Add butter, milk, salt, and pepper, and mash until smooth.

6. Serve the stroganoff over the mashed cauliflower.

Nutritional Values (per serving):
Calories: 250 | Fat: 12g | Cholesterol: 15mg |
Carbs: 30g | Fiber: 7g | Protein: 8g |
Sodium: 550mg

Cauliflower Fried Rice

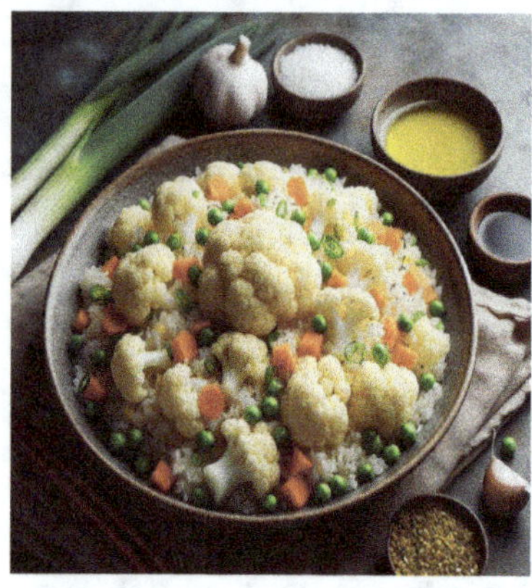

Preparation Time: 15 minutes
Cooking Time: 15 minutes
Servings: 4

Ingredients:
- 1 head cauliflower (grated)
- 2 tablespoons vegetable oil
- 1 onion (diced)
- 2 carrots (diced)
- 1 cup peas (frozen)
- 2 cloves garlic (minced)
- - 2 eggs (beaten)
- 3 tablespoons soy sauce
- 1 teaspoon sesame oil
- Green onions for garnish

Directions:
1. In a large wok or skillet, heat vegetable oil over medium-high heat.

2. Add diced onion, diced carrots, and frozen peas. Stir-fry until vegetables are tender.

3. Push vegetables to one side of the wok and pour beaten eggs into the empty space. Scramble the eggs until cooked.

4. Mix in the grated cauliflower, minced garlic, soy sauce, and sesame oil. Stir-fry for 5-7 minutes until cauliflower is cooked through.

5. Garnish with sliced green onions before serving.

Nutritional Values (per serving):
Calories: 180 | Fat: 10g | Cholesterol: 95mg |
Carbs: 18g | Fiber: 7g | Protein: 9g |
Sodium: 700mg

Broccoli Beef Stir-Fry

Preparation Time: 15 minutes
Cooking Time: 15 minutes
Servings: 4

Ingredients:
- 1 lb flank steak (sliced thinly)
- 1/4 cup soy sauce
- 2 tablespoons oyster sauce
- 1 tablespoon hoisin sauce
- 1 tablespoon cornstarch
- 2 tablespoons vegetable oil
- 4 cups broccoli florets
- 2 cloves garlic (minced)
- 1 tablespoon ginger (minced)
- Cooked rice for serving

Directions:
1. In a bowl, marinate sliced flank steak in soy sauce, oyster sauce, hoisin sauce, and cornstarch. Give it ten minutes or more to sit.
2. In a wok or large skillet, heat the vegetable oil over high heat.
3. Add marinated beef to the wok and stir-fry until browned. Take out of the wok and place aside..

4. In the same wok, stir-fry broccoli florets, minced garlic, and minced ginger until broccoli is tender-crisp.

5. Add the cooked beef back to the wok and toss until everything is well coated.

6. Serve the broccoli beef stir-fry over cooked rice.

Nutritional Values (per serving):
Calories: 350 | Fat: 15g | Cholesterol: 45mg |
Carbs: 20g | Fiber: 4g | Protein: 30g |
Sodium: 950mg

Pork Chops and Applesauce

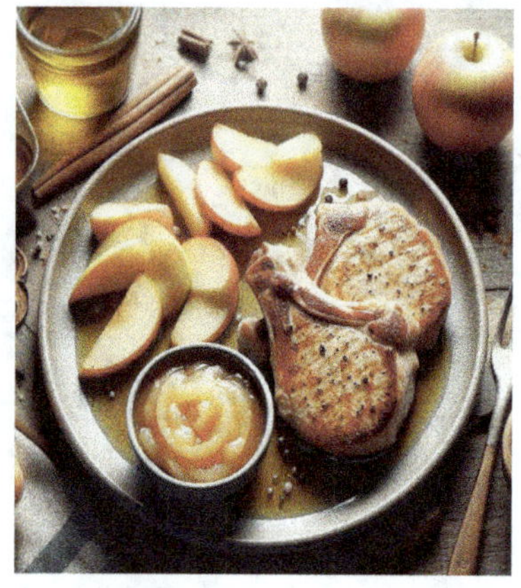

Preparation Time: 10 minutes
Cooking Time: 20 minutes
Servings: 4

Ingredients:
- 4 pork chops
- Salt and pepper to taste
- 2 tablespoons olive oil
- 2 apples (peeled, cored, and sliced)
- 1 tablespoon butter
- 1 tablespoon brown sugar
- 1/2 teaspoon cinnamon
- 1/4 cup apple cider or apple juice

Directions:
1. Season pork chops with salt and pepper.

2. In a large skillet, heat olive oil over medium-high heat. Add pork chops and cook until browned on both sides and cooked through.

3. In a separate pan, melt butter and sauté apple slices until softened.

4. Stir in brown sugar, cinnamon, and apple cider. Cook until apples are caramelized.

5. Serve the pork chops with a generous spoonful of applesauce.

Nutritional Values (per serving):
Calories: 350 | Fat: 18g | Cholesterol: 90mg |
Carbs: 22g | Fiber: 3g | Protein: 25g |
Sodium: 80mg

Creamy Broccoli Soup

Preparation Time: 15 minutes
Cooking Time: 25 minutes
Servings: 6

Ingredients:
- 4 cups broccoli florets
- 1 onion (chopped)
- 2 carrots (chopped)
- 3 cups vegetable broth
- 2 cups milk (any type)
- 3 tablespoons flour
- 2 tablespoons butter
- 1/2 teaspoon garlic powder
- Salt and pepper to taste
- Shredded cheddar cheese for garnish (optional)

Directions:
1. Melt butter in a big saucepan over a medium heat. Cook the chopped onion until it becomes tender.
2. Stir in flour to create a roux, then gradually whisk in vegetable broth until smooth.

3. Add chopped carrots, broccoli florets, garlic powder, salt, and pepper. Simmer until vegetables are tender.

4. Smoothly purée the soup using an immersion blender.

5. Pour in milk, stirring constantly, and continue to simmer until heated through.

6. Adjust seasoning if necessary. Serve hot, optionally garnished with shredded cheddar cheese.

Nutritional Values (per serving):
**Calories: 180 | Fat: 10g | Cholesterol: 20mg |
Carbs: 18g | Fiber: 4g | Protein: 8g |
Sodium: 550mg**

Chicken Noodle Soup

Preparation Time: 15 minutes
Cooking Time: 30 minutes
Servings: 6

Ingredients:
- 1 lb chicken breasts (cooked and shredded)
- 8 cups chicken broth
- 2 carrots (sliced)
- 2 celery stalks (sliced)
- 1 onion (chopped)
- 2 cloves garlic (minced)
- 2 cups egg noodles
- 1 teaspoon dried thyme
- Salt and pepper to taste
- Fresh parsley for garnish

Directions:
1. In a large pot, combine chicken broth, sliced carrots, sliced celery, chopped onion, and minced garlic.
2. Bring to a boil, then reduce heat and simmer until vegetables are tender.
3. Add shredded chicken, egg noodles, dried thyme, salt, and pepper. Cook until noodles are tender.

4. Adjust seasoning if necessary. Garnish with fresh parsley before serving.

Nutritional Values (per serving):
Calories: 250 | Fat: 5g | Cholesterol: 50mg |
Carbs: 20g | Fiber: 2g | Protein: 30g |
Sodium: 750mg

Honey-Glazed Salmon

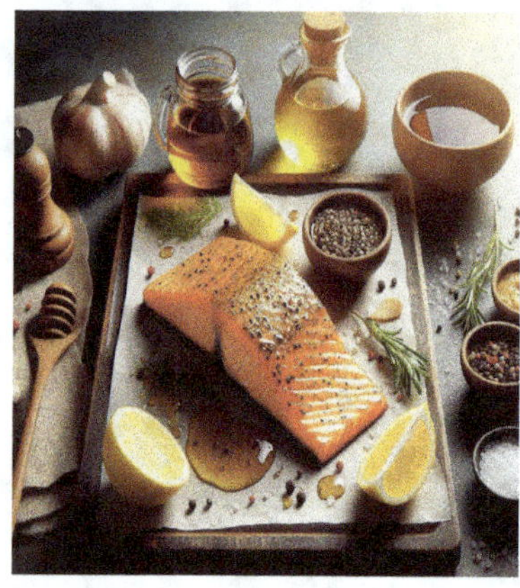

Preparation Time: 10 minutes
Cooking Time: 15 minutes
Servings: 2

Ingredients:
- 2 salmon fillets
- 2 tablespoons honey
- 1 tablespoon soy sauce
- 1 tablespoon Dijon mustard
- 1 teaspoon minced garlic
- Salt and pepper to taste
- Fresh lemon wedges for serving

Directions:
1. Preheat the oven to 400°F (200°C).
2. In a small bowl, whisk together honey, soy sauce,
Dijon mustard, minced garlic, salt, and pepper.

3. Place salmon fillets on a baking sheet and brush the glaze over the top.

4. Bake for 15 minutes or until salmon is cooked through and flaky.

5. Serve with fresh lemon wedges.

Nutritional Values (per serving):
Calories: 320 | Fat: 15g | Cholesterol: 75mg |
Carbs: 18g | Fiber: 0g | Protein: 30g |
Sodium: 550mg

Zucchini Noodles

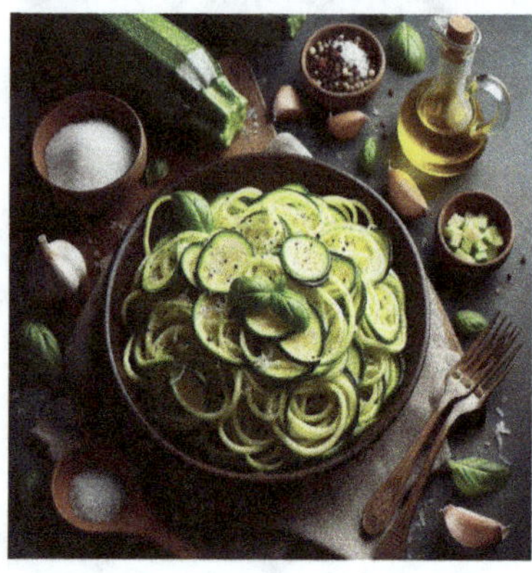

Preparation Time: 10 minutes
Cooking Time: 5 minutes
Servings: 4

Ingredients:
- 4 medium zucchinis
- 2 tablespoons olive oil
- 2 cloves garlic (minced)
- Salt and pepper to taste
- Grated Parmesan cheese for garnish (optional)
- Chopped fresh basil for garnish

Directions:
1. Spiralize the zucchinis to make noodles out of them.
2. In a big skillet over medium heat, warm up the olive oil. Sauté the minced garlic for one to two minutes.

3. Add zucchini noodles to the skillet and toss until heated through but still crisp.

4. Season with salt and pepper to taste.

5. Optional: Garnish with grated Parmesan cheese and chopped fresh basil.

Nutritional Values (per serving):
Calories: 80 | Fat: 7g | Cholesterol: 0mg |
Carbs: 4g | Fiber: 2g | Protein: 2g |
Sodium: 10mg

Spinach Salad with Shrimps

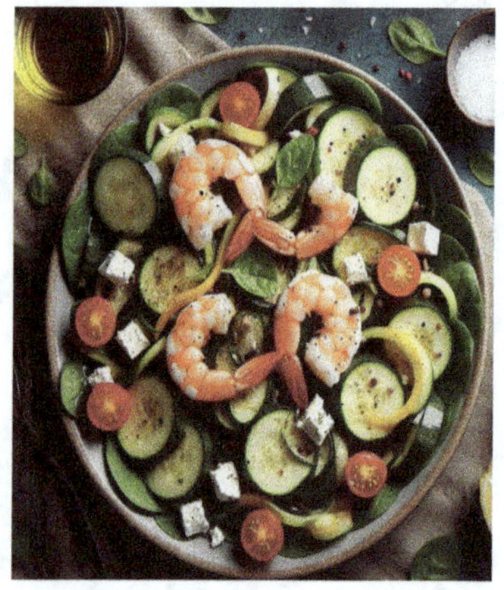

Preparation Time: 15 minutes
Cooking Time: 5 minutes
Servings: 2

Ingredients:
- 2 cups fresh spinach leaves
- 1/2 lb shrimp (cooked and peeled)
- 1 cup cherry tomatoes (halved)
- 1/2 cucumber (sliced)
- 1/4 cup feta cheese (crumbled)
- 2 tablespoons olive oil
- 1 tablespoon balsamic vinegar
- Salt and pepper to taste

Directions:

1. In a large bowl, combine fresh spinach leaves, cooked shrimp, cherry tomatoes, sliced cucumber, and crumbled feta cheese.

2. Mix the balsamic vinegar and olive oil in a small bowl. Drizzle over the salad.

3. Toss the salad until well coated. Season with salt and pepper to taste.

4. Serve immediately.

Nutritional Values (per serving):
Calories: 320 | Fat: 20g | Cholesterol: 120mg |
Carbs: 18g | Fiber: 4g | Protein: 20g |
Sodium: 450mg

Baked Salmon Steaks

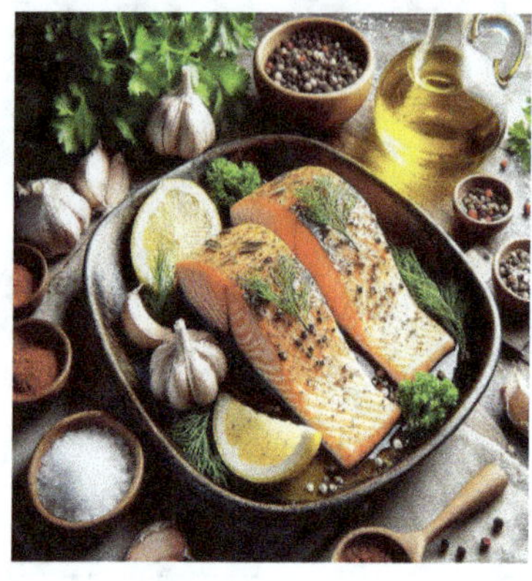

Preparation Time: 15 minutes
Cooking Time: 20 minutes
Servings: 2

Ingredients:
- 2 salmon steaks
- 2 tablespoons olive oil
- 1 lemon (juiced)
- Salt and pepper to taste
- 1 teaspoon dried dill
- 1 teaspoon paprika
- 2 cloves garlic (minced)
- Fresh parsley for garnish

Directions:
1. Preheat the oven to 400°F (200°C).
2. Place salmon steaks on a baking sheet lined with parchment paper.

3. In a small bowl, mix olive oil, lemon juice, salt, pepper, dried dill, paprika, and minced garlic.
4. Brush the olive oil mixture over the salmon steaks, ensuring they are well coated.
5. Bake for 20 minutes or until the salmon is cooked through and flakes easily.
6. Garnish with fresh parsley before serving.

Nutritional Values (per serving):
Calories: 350 | Fat: 20g | Cholesterol: 80mg | Carbs: 2g | Fiber: 0g | Protein: 30g | Sodium: 450mg

---

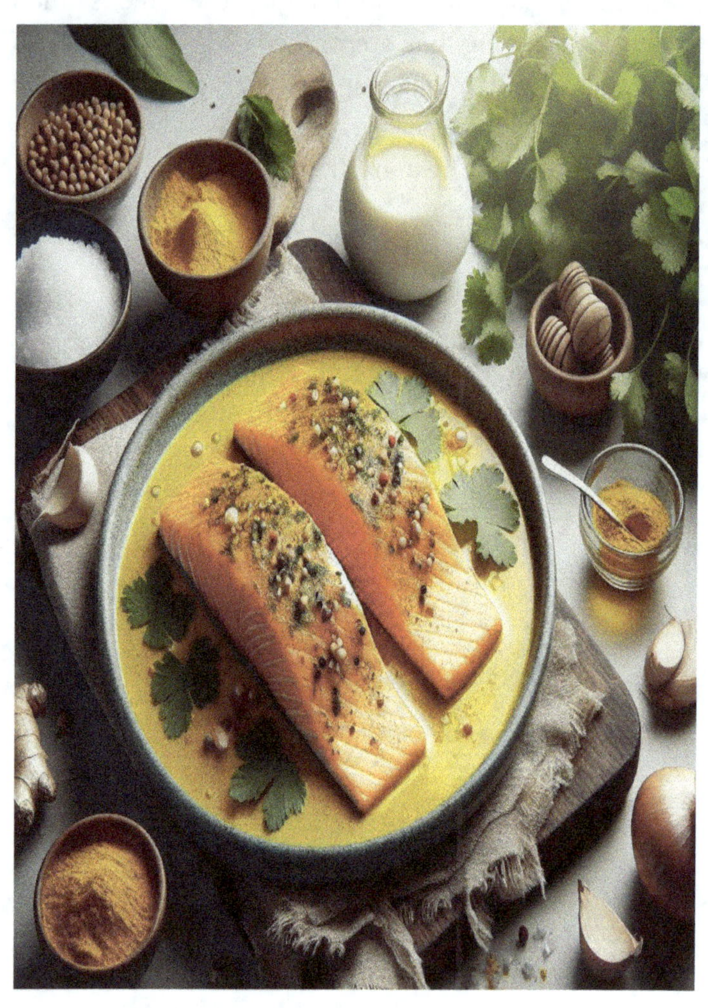

Chapter 7: Desserts/Snacks

Quick-Roasted Cauliflower

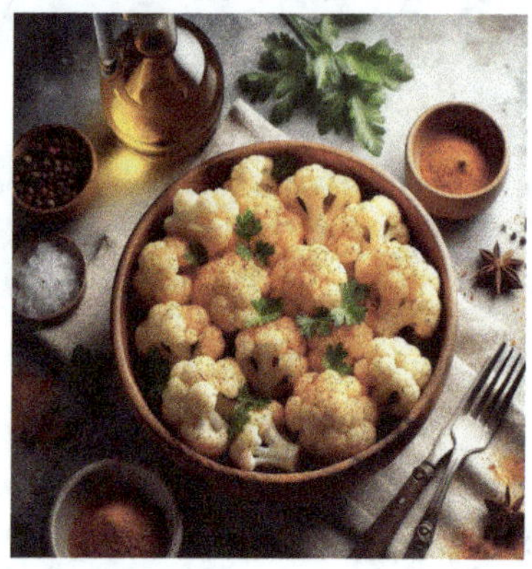

Preparation Time: 10 minutes
Cooking Time: 20 minutes
Servings: 4

Ingredients:
- 1 head cauliflower (cut into florets)
- 2 tablespoons olive oil
- 1 teaspoon cumin
- 1 teaspoon paprika
- 1/2 teaspoon garlic powder
- Salt and pepper to taste
- Fresh parsley for garnish

Directions:
1. Preheat the oven to 425°F (220°C).
2. In a large bowl, toss cauliflower florets with olive oil, cumin, paprika, garlic powder, salt, and pepper until well coated.

3. Spread the cauliflower on a baking sheet in a single layer.

4. Roast for 20 minutes or until the cauliflower is golden and tender.

5. Garnish with fresh parsley before serving.

Nutritional Values (per serving):
Calories: 120 | Fat: 7g | Cholesterol: 0mg |
Carbs: 14g | Fiber: 5g | Protein: 4g |
Sodium: 150mg

Chocolate Fudge Cake

Preparation Time: 15 minutes
Cooking Time: 30 minutes
Servings: 8

Ingredients:
- 1 cup all-purpose flour
- 1 cup granulated sugar
- 1/2 cup unsweetened cocoa powder
- 1 teaspoon baking powder
- 1/2 teaspoon baking soda
- 1/2 teaspoon salt
- 1/2 cup milk
- 1/4 cup vegetable oil
- 2 large eggs
- 2 teaspoons vanilla extract
- 1/2 cup boiling water
- Powdered sugar for dusting (optional)

Directions:
1. Preheat the oven to 350°F (180°C). Grease and flour a cake pan.
2. Mix the flour, sugar, baking soda, cocoa powder, baking powder, and salt in a big basin.

3. Include the eggs, milk, vegetable oil, and vanilla essence. Mix until well combined.

4. Stir in boiling water until the batter is smooth. The batter will be thin.

5. Pour the batter into the prepared cake pan and bake for 30 minutes or until a toothpick inserted into the center comes out clean.

6. Allow the cake to cool completely before dusting with powdered sugar if desired.

Nutritional Values (per serving):
Calories: 280 | Fat: 10g | Cholesterol: 45mg |
Carbs: 45g | Fiber: 3g | Protein: 5g |
Sodium: 250mg

Walnut Cheesecake

Preparation Time: 20 minutes
Cooking Time: 50 minutes
Servings: 10

Ingredients:
For the Crust:
- 1½ cups graham cracker crumbs
- 1/2 cup melted butter
- 1/4 cup granulated sugar

For the Filling:
- 3 packets (24 ounces) softened cream cheese
- 1 cup granulated sugar
- 1 teaspoon vanilla extract
- 3 large eggs
- 1/2 cup sour cream
- 1/2 cup chopped walnuts

Directions:
1. Preheat the oven to 325°F (160°C). Grease a springform pan.
2. In a bowl, combine graham cracker crumbs, melted butter, and granulated sugar. Press firmly onto the pan's bottom.

3. In a large bowl, beat softened cream cheese, sugar, and vanilla extract until smooth.

4. Gently whisk in each egg as you add it, one at a time. Stir in sour cream and chopped walnuts.

5. Pour the cream cheese mixture over the crust.

6. Bake for 50 minutes, or until the middle/center sets.

7. Allow the cheesecake to cool in the pan, then refrigerate for at least 4 hours or overnight before serving.

Nutritional Values (per serving):
Calories: 450 | Fat: 30g | Cholesterol: 120mg |
Carbs: 40g | Fiber: 1g | Protein: 8g |
Sodium: 350mg

Easy Chocolate Mousse

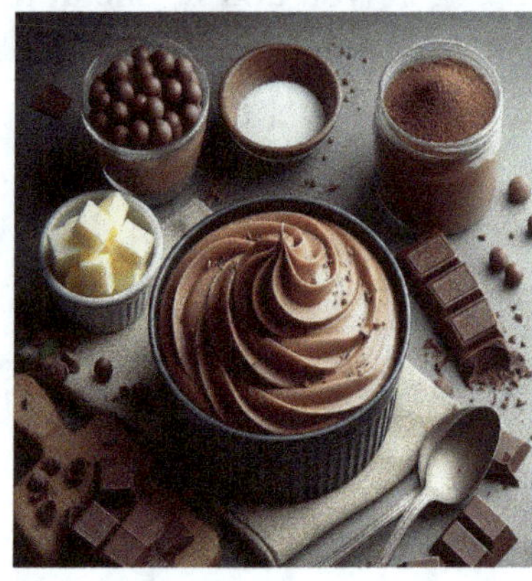

Preparation Time: 15 minutes
Chilling Time: 2 hours
Servings: 6

Ingredients:
- 1 cup semi-sweet chocolate chips
- 2 tablespoons unsalted butter
- 2 cups heavy cream
- 1/4 cup powdered sugar
- 1 teaspoon vanilla extract
- Chocolate shavings for garnish (optional)

Directions:
1. In a heatproof bowl, melt chocolate chips and butter together. Allow to cool slightly.
2. Beat heavy cream in a separate basin until soft peaks form. Add the vanilla extract and powdered sugar and continue beating until firm peaks form.

3. Gently fold the melted chocolate mixture into the whipped cream until well combined.

4. Divide the mousse into serving glasses and refrigerate for at least 2 hours.

5. Garnish with chocolate shavings before serving.

Nutritional Values (per serving):
**Calories: 350 | Fat: 30g | Cholesterol: 90mg |
Carbs: 20g | Fiber: 2g | Protein: 3g |
Sodium: 30mg**

Butternut Spice Cookies

Preparation Time: 15 minutes
Cooking Time: 12 minutes
Servings: 24 cookies

Ingredients:
- 1 cup unsalted butter (softened)
- 1 cup granulated sugar
- 1 cup brown sugar (packed)
- 2 large eggs
- 1 teaspoon vanilla extract
- 2 cups all-purpose flour
- 1 teaspoon baking soda
- 1/2 teaspoon baking powder
- 1/2 teaspoon salt
- 1 teaspoon ground cinnamon
- 1/2 teaspoon ground nutmeg
- 1/2 teaspoon ground ginger
- 1/4 teaspoon ground cloves
- 2 cups butternut squash (grated)
- 1 cup rolled oats

Directions:
1. Preheat the oven to 350°F (180°C). Line baking sheets with parchment paper.

2. Beat softened butter, brown sugar, and granulated sugar in a large bowl until frothy and light.

3. Beat thoroughly after adding each egg, one at a time. Stir in vanilla extract.

4. In a separate bowl, whisk together flour, baking soda, baking powder, salt, cinnamon, nutmeg, ginger, and cloves.

5. Add the dry ingredients to the wet ingredients gradually and stir until well blended.

6. Fold in grated butternut squash and rolled oats.

7. Drop rounded tablespoons of dough onto the prepared baking sheets.

8. Bake for 12 minutes, or until golden brown around the edges.

9. Let the cookies cool for a few minutes on the baking sheets, then move them to a wire rack to finish cooling.

Nutritional Values (per serving - 1 cookie):
Calories: 160 | Fat: 7g | Cholesterol: 30mg |
Carbs: 23g | Fiber: 1g | Protein: 2g |
Sodium: 90mg

Creamy Chocolate Avocado Pudding

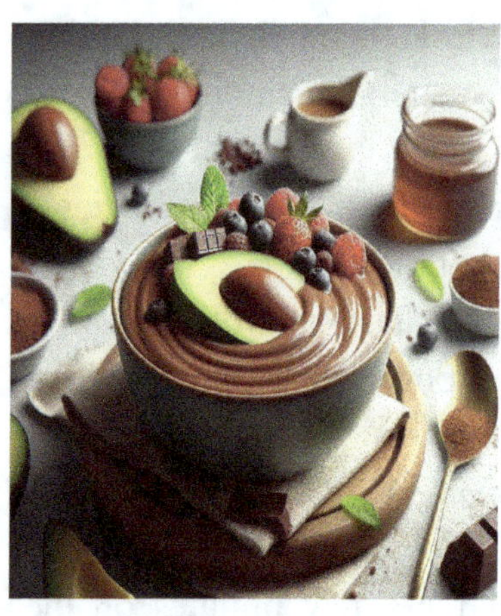

Preparation Time: 10 minutes
Chilling Time: 2 hours
Servings: 4

Ingredients:
- 2 ripe avocados
- 1/4 cup cocoa powder
- 1/4 cup honey or maple syrup
- 1/4 cup milk (any type)
- 1 teaspoon vanilla extract
- A pinch of salt
- Fresh berries for garnish

Directions:
1. In a blender or food processor, combine ripe avocados, cocoa powder, honey or maple syrup, milk, vanilla extract, and a pinch of salt.

2. Blend until smooth and creamy.

3. Transfer the pudding to serving bowls and refrigerate for at least 2 hours.

4. Garnish with fresh berries before serving.

Nutritional Values (per serving):
Calories: 220 | Fat: 15g | Cholesterol: 0mg |
Carbs: 25g | Fiber: 7g | Protein: 3g |
Sodium: 10mg

Bean Dip with Tortilla Chips

Preparation Time: 15 minutes
Cooking Time: 10 minutes
Servings: 6

Ingredients:
- 2 cans (15 oz each) washed and drained black beans
- 1/4 cup olive oil
- 2 cloves garlic (minced)
- 1 teaspoon cumin
- 1/2 teaspoon chili powder
- 1/4 teaspoon cayenne pepper
- Salt and pepper to taste
- 1/4 cup fresh cilantro (chopped)
- 1 lime (juiced)
- Tortilla chips for serving

Directions:
1. In a food processor, combine black beans, olive oil, minced garlic, cumin, chili powder, cayenne pepper, salt, and pepper.
2. Blend until smooth, adding more olive oil if needed.
3. Transfer the bean dip to a serving bowl.

4. Stir in chopped cilantro and lime juice.
5. Serve with tortilla chips.

91

Strawberry Granita

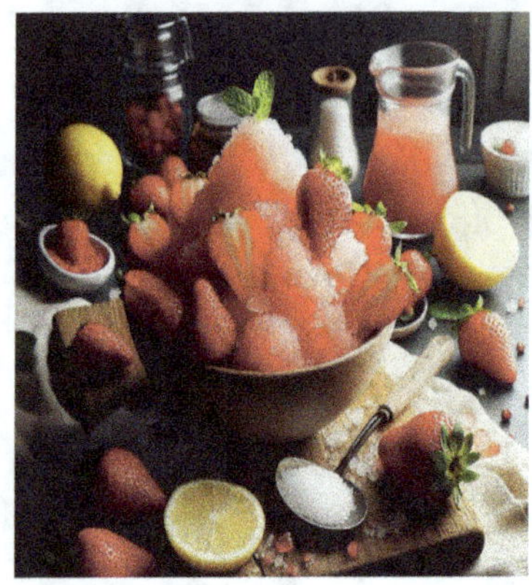

Preparation Time: 10 minutes
Freezing Time: 6 hours
Servings: 4

Ingredients:
- 1 lb fresh strawberries (hulled)
- 1/2 cup granulated sugar
- 1/4 cup water
- 1 tablespoon fresh lemon juice

Directions:
1. In a blender, combine fresh strawberries and granulated sugar.
2. Blend until smooth.
3. In a saucepan, heat water over medium heat until sugar dissolves, creating a simple syrup.
4. Add the strawberry puree and fresh lemon juice to the simple syrup. Stir well.

5. After transferring the mixture to a shallow dish, freeze it.

6. Every 30 minutes, scrape the granita with a fork to create a flaky texture.

7. Continue freezing and scraping until the granita is fully frozen and has a shaved ice consistency.

8. Serve in chilled glasses.

Nutritional Values (per serving):
Calories: 100 | Fat: 0g | Cholesterol: 0mg |
Carbs: 26g | Fiber: 3g | Protein: 1g |
Sodium: 0mg

Fermented Cauliflower Pickles

Preparation Time: 20 minutes
Fermentation Time: 5-7 days
Servings: 1 large jar

Ingredients:
- 1 large cauliflower head (cut into florets)
- 3 cloves garlic (sliced)
- 1 tablespoon mustard seeds
- 1 tablespoon black peppercorns
- 1 teaspoon red pepper flakes
- 2-3 bay leaves
- Brine solution (1 quart water mixed with 2 tablespoons sea salt)

Directions:
1. Sterilize a large glass jar.
2. In the jar, layer cauliflower florets, sliced garlic, mustard seeds, black peppercorns, red pepper flakes, and bay leaves.
3. Prepare the brine solution by dissolving sea salt in water.
4. Pour the brine solution over the cauliflower, ensuring it fully covers the vegetables.

5. Place a weight (like a smaller jar filled with water) on top to keep the cauliflower submerged.

6. Cover the jar loosely and place it in a cool, dark place for 5-7 days, checking for desired fermentation taste.

7. Once fermented, store the cauliflower pickles in the refrigerator.

Nutritional Values (per serving):
Calories: 20 | Fat: 0g | Cholesterol: 0mg |
Carbs: 4g | Fiber: 2g | Protein: 1g |
Sodium: 2500mg

Slow-Cooked Collard Greens

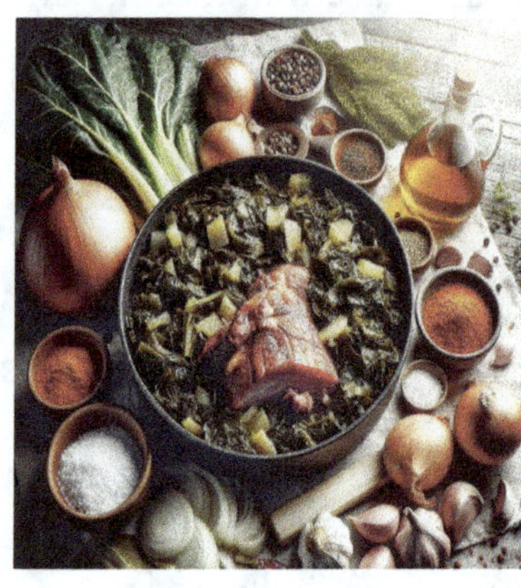

Preparation Time: 15 minutes
Cooking Time: 4-6 hours
Servings: 6

Ingredients:
- 2 bunches collard greens (washed and chopped)
- 1 onion (chopped)
- 3 cloves garlic (minced)
- 1 smoked ham hock or turkey neck
- 1 teaspoon red pepper flakes
- 1 teaspoon smoked paprika
- 1 teaspoon apple cider vinegar
- Salt and pepper to taste

Directions:

1. In a slow cooker, combine collard greens, chopped onion, minced garlic, smoked ham hock or turkey neck, red pepper flakes, smoked paprika, apple cider vinegar, salt, and pepper.

2. Cook on low for 4-6 hours until the collard greens are tender.

3. Before serving, remove the ham hock or turkey neck and shred the meat.

4. Stir the shredded meat back into the collard greens and adjust seasoning if necessary.

Nutritional Values (per serving):
**Calories: 120 | Fat: 2g | Cholesterol: 10mg |
Carbs: 20g | Fiber: 8g | Protein: 6g |
Sodium: 350mg**

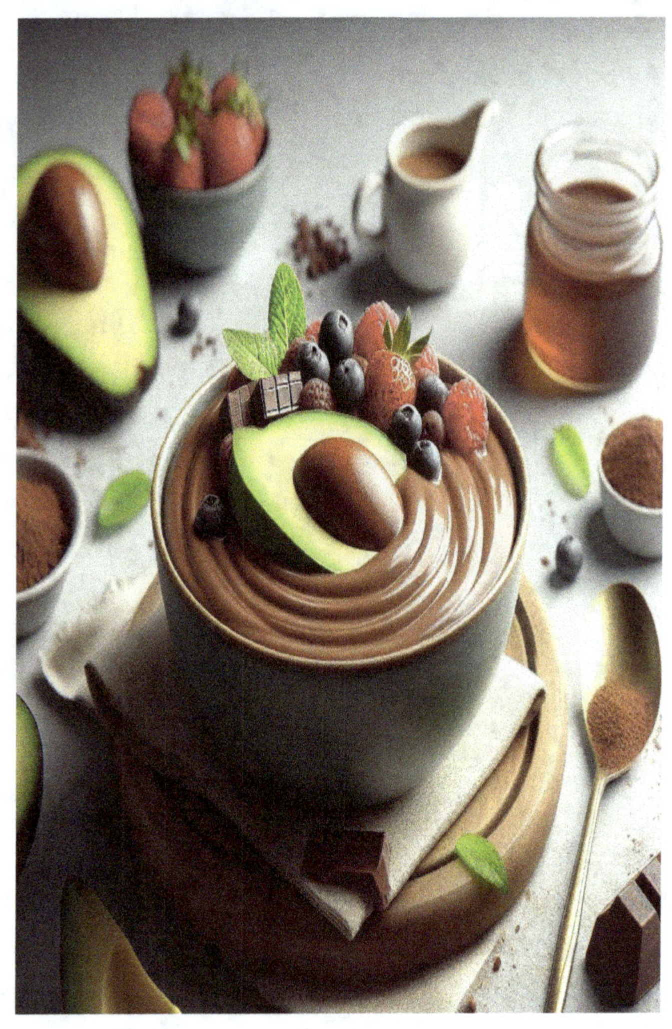

Chapter 8: Meal Planning and Grocery Shopping Tips

Living with Lupus often means balancing busy schedules with the demands of managing your health. Cooking nutritious and delicious meals can feel like a daunting task, but with smart planning and savvy shopping strategies, you can conquer the kitchen with confidence and create a Lupus-friendly feast!

Mastering the Meal Plan

- **Weekly Roadmap**: Dedicate a day to plan your meals for the week. Consider your schedule, energy levels, and any Lupus flares you might be experiencing.
- **Variety is Key**: Rotate your protein sources, explore different vegetables, and experiment with whole grains to avoid dietary boredom and ensure nutritional balance.
- **Leftovers are Lifesavers**: Cook larger batches at the weekend and portion them out for easy weekday lunches or dinners.
- **Slow Cooker & Instant Pot Magic**: Utilize these time-saving kitchen appliances to prepare slow-cooked stews, soups, and healthy one-pot meals.

- **Don't Forget Breakfast**: This meal sets the tone for your day. Prepare quick and easy options like overnight oats, chia pudding, or veggie scrambled eggs for busy mornings.

Grocery Shopping Smarts

- **Make a List & Stick to It**: Plan your meals before stepping into the grocery store to avoid impulse buys and unhealthy temptations.
- **Shop the Perimeter First**: Fill your cart with fresh produce, lean protein, and whole grains first. These healthy staples should make up the bulk of your purchases.
- **Read Food Labels**: Be mindful of added sugars, saturated fats, and sodium. Choose foods with short ingredient lists and prioritize natural whole foods.
- **Stock Up on Staples**: Keep pantry essentials like canned beans, lentils, brown rice, and quinoa on hand for quick and nutritious meals.
- **Freeze for Convenience**: Portion and freeze healthy recipes for future convenience. This is especially helpful when Lupus flares limit your energy levels.
- **Don't Be Afraid to Ask for Help**: Utilize grocery store delivery services or delegate

shopping tasks to loved ones when fatigue hits.

Beyond the Basics

- **Make it a Family Affair**: Get your family involved in meal planning and cooking. This can be a fun bonding experience and a way to educate everyone about Lupus-friendly choices.
- **Batch Your Prep**: Chop vegetables, marinate meats, and cook grains in advance to save time on busy weeknights.
- **Utilize Leftovers Creatively**: Repurpose leftover ingredients into new dishes. Leftover roasted chicken can become a salad topping, and cooked grains can form the base for stir-fries or stuffed peppers.
- **Keep it Simple**: Don't overcomplicate things. Simple, one-pan meals or sheet pan dinners are healthy and require minimal cleanup.
- **Celebrate Small Victories**: Cooking nutritious meals for yourself is a victory! Be proud of your efforts and focus on progress, not perfection.

Remember, conquering the kitchen with Lupus is all about making choices that work for you. By planning, shopping smart, and adapting recipes to your needs, you can create delicious and nutritious meals that fuel your body and support your well-being. Let your kitchen become a space of creativity, nourishment, and self-care, where you nourish not just your body, but also your spirit and sense of accomplishment. Bon appétit!

14-Day Meal Plan

Day 1:
Breakfast: Coconut Banana Breakfast Cookies
Lunch: Balsamic Vinaigrette Veggie Burrito Bowl
Dinner: Mushroom Stroganoff over Mashed Cauliflower
Snack/Dessert: Quick-Roasted Cauliflower

Day 2:
Breakfast: Chia Seed Pudding
Lunch: Turmeric Coconut Salmon
Dinner: Cauliflower Fried Rice
Snack/Dessert: Chocolate Fudge Cake

Day 3:
Breakfast: Hearty Blueberry Pancakes
Lunch: Easy Avocado Egg Salad Cucumber Sandwiches
Dinner: Broccoli Beef Stir-Fry
Snack/Dessert: Walnut Cheesecake

Day 4:
Breakfast: Chocolate Banana Smoothie
Lunch: Bean and Rice Salad
Dinner: Pork Chops and Applesauce
Snack/Dessert: Easy Chocolate Mousse

Day 5:
Breakfast: Breakfast Burrito Bowl
Lunch: Italian Poached Sea Bass
Dinner: Creamy Broccoli Soup
Snack/Dessert: Butternut Spice Cookies

Day 6:
Breakfast: Cauliflower Hash Browns
Lunch: Slow Cooker Carnitas
Dinner: Chicken Noodle Soup
Snack/Dessert: Creamy Chocolate Avocado Pudding

Day 7:
Breakfast: Grain-Free Pumpkin Pancakes
Lunch: Butternut Squash Soup Vegetable Stir-Fry
Dinner: Honey-Glazed Salmon
Snack/Dessert: Bean Dip with Tortilla Chips

Day 8:

Breakfast: Butternut Squash Porridge
Lunch: Mushroom Stroganoff over Mashed Cauliflower
Dinner: Zucchini Noodles
Snack/Dessert: Strawberry Granita

Day 9:

Breakfast: Sweet Potato, Kale, and Mushroom Scramble
Lunch: Cauliflower Fried Rice
Dinner: Spinach Salad with Shrimps
Snack/Dessert: Fermented Cauliflower Pickles

Day 10:

Breakfast: Coconut Pudding
Lunch: Balsamic Vinaigrette Veggie Burrito Bowl
Dinner: Baked Salmon Steaks
Snack/Dessert: Slow-Cooked Collard Greens

Day 11:

Breakfast: Chocolate Banana Smoothie
Lunch: Italian Poached Sea Bass
Dinner: Broccoli Beef Stir-Fry
Snack/Dessert: Walnut Cheesecake

Day 12:
Breakfast: Hearty Blueberry Pancakes
Lunch: Easy Avocado Egg Salad Cucumber Sandwiches
Dinner: Creamy Broccoli Soup
Snack/Dessert: Chocolate Fudge Cake

Day 13:
Breakfast: Breakfast Burrito Bowl
Lunch: Slow Cooker Carnitas
Dinner: Chicken Noodle Soup
Snack/Dessert: Easy Chocolate Mousse

Day 14:
Breakfast: Grain-Free Pumpkin Pancakes
Lunch: Butternut Squash Soup Vegetable Stir-Fry
Dinner: Honey-Glazed Salmon
Snack/Dessert: Strawberry Granita

Feel free to repeat or mix and match based on your preferences. Adjust portions according to your dietary needs and consult with a nutritionist if necessary. Enjoy your 14-day meal plan!

Conclusion

You flipped the final page, the taste of victory lingering on your tongue like the last burst of ginger in a stir-fry. This book, once a lifeline, now sits closed, a trophy on your kitchen counter. The pantry, once sparsely stocked, groans with colorful rebellion. Your fridge, no longer a battlefield, hums with the quiet confidence of a well-armed arsenal.

Lupus is still there, lurking in the shadows, waiting for its chance to pounce. But you? You're different now. You've tasted the fiery defiance of turmeric, the sunshine resilience of lemon, the comforting strength of bone broth. You've learned to dance with inflammation, to laugh in the face of fatigue, to wage war with every bite.

Remember, this journey wasn't a sprint, it was a slow simmer, a patient dance with your body. There were days when the flames sputtered, when doubt tasted like burnt toast. But you rebuilt, brick by flavorful brick, fuelled by the memory of Aunt Marie's salsa-fueled spirit.

Now, stand tall, warrior. You've faced the lupus beast, not with a whimper, but with a well-seasoned wok and a rebellious grin. You've learned to cook your way back to life, one delicious victory at a time. Go forth, share your story, your recipes, your hard-won wisdom. Show the world that a diagnosis isn't a destiny, it's just another spice in the grand, delicious pot of life.

So cook on, my friend. Let your kitchen be a weapon of joy, your meals a symphony of defiance. Remember, every flare-up is just a chance to reinvent your dish, every setback a call to add a new, bolder flavor. You are more than Lupus, more than any diagnosis. You are the chef, the artist, the alchemist of your own life. Keep stirring, keep tasting, keep dancing. Your best recipe is yet to be written.

Now, close your eyes, take a deep breath, and savor the sweet, spicy heat of triumph. You did it. And you can do it again. Every damn time.

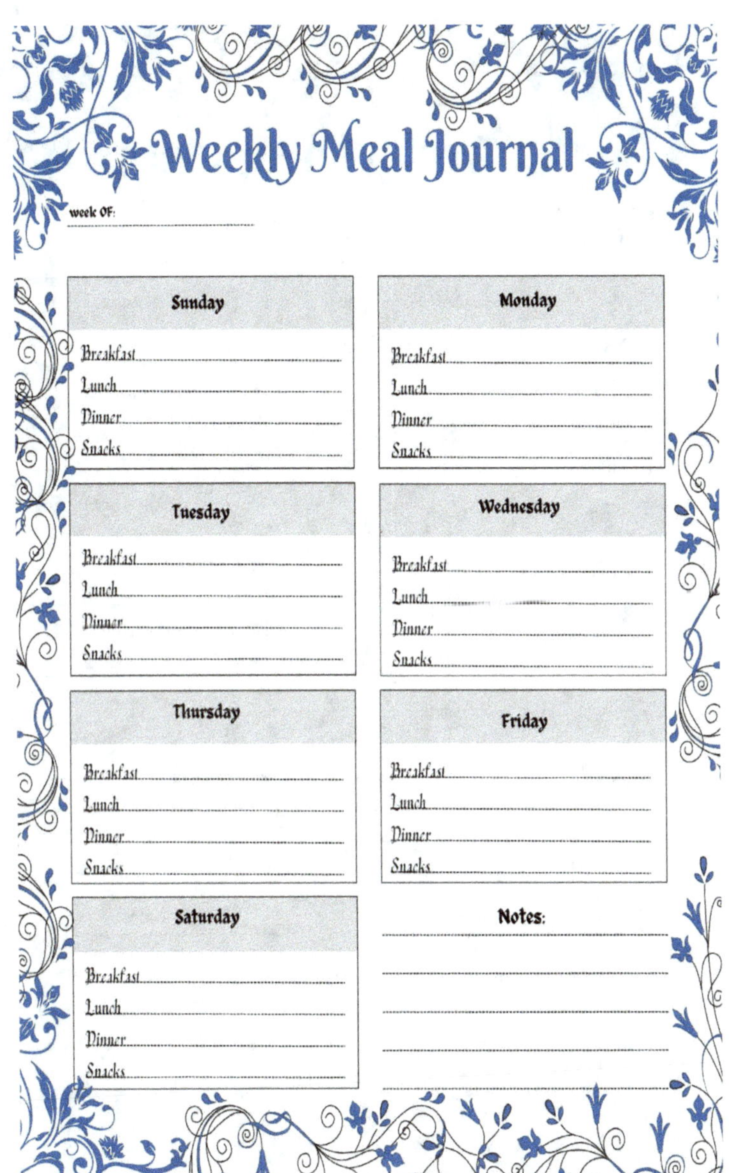

Weekly Meal Journal
week OF:

Sunday
Breakfast
Lunch
Dinner
Snacks

Monday
Breakfast
Lunch
Dinner
Snacks

Tuesday
Breakfast
Lunch
Dinner
Snacks

Wednesday
Breakfast
Lunch
Dinner
Snacks

Thursday
Breakfast
Lunch
Dinner
Snacks

Friday
Breakfast
Lunch
Dinner
Snacks

Saturday
Breakfast
Lunch
Dinner
Snacks

Notes:

Weekly Meal Journal

week OF: _______________

Sunday

Breakfast ....
Lunch ....
Dinner ....
Snacks ....

Monday

Breakfast ....
Lunch ....
Dinner ....
Snacks ....

Tuesday

Breakfast ....
Lunch ....
Dinner ....
Snacks ....

Wednesday

Breakfast ....
Lunch ....
Dinner ....
Snacks ....

Thursday

Breakfast ....
Lunch ....
Dinner ....
Snacks ....

Friday

Breakfast ....
Lunch ....
Dinner ....
Snacks ....

Saturday

Breakfast ....
Lunch ....
Dinner ....
Snacks ....

Notes:

....

....

....

Weekly Meal Journal

week OF: ....

Sunday

Breakfast ....
Lunch ....
Dinner ....
Snacks ....

Monday

Breakfast ....
Lunch ....
Dinner ....
Snacks ....

Tuesday

Breakfast ....
Lunch ....
Dinner ....
Snacks ....

Wednesday

Breakfast ....
Lunch ....
Dinner ....
Snacks ....

Thursday

Breakfast ....
Lunch ....
Dinner ....
Snacks ....

Friday

Breakfast ....
Lunch ....
Dinner ....
Snacks ....

Saturday

Breakfast ....
Lunch ....
Dinner ....
Snacks ....

Notes:

Weekly Meal Journal

week OF: _______________

Sunday

Breakfast _______________
Lunch _______________
Dinner _______________
Snacks _______________

Monday

Breakfast _______________
Lunch _______________
Dinner _______________
Snacks _______________

Tuesday

Breakfast _______________
Lunch _______________
Dinner _______________
Snacks _______________

Wednesday

Breakfast _______________
Lunch _______________
Dinner _______________
Snacks _______________

Thursday

Breakfast _______________
Lunch _______________
Dinner _______________
Snacks _______________

Friday

Breakfast _______________
Lunch _______________
Dinner _______________
Snacks _______________

Saturday

Breakfast _______________
Lunch _______________
Dinner _______________
Snacks _______________

Notes:

____
____
____
____

Weekly Meal Journal

week OF: _______________________

Sunday

Breakfast ___________________________
Lunch ___________________________
Dinner ___________________________
Snacks ___________________________

Monday

Breakfast ___________________________
Lunch ___________________________
Dinner ___________________________
Snacks ___________________________

Tuesday

Breakfast ___________________________
Lunch ___________________________
Dinner ___________________________
Snacks ___________________________

Wednesday

Breakfast ___________________________
Lunch ___________________________
Dinner ___________________________
Snacks ___________________________

Thursday

Breakfast ___________________________
Lunch ___________________________
Dinner ___________________________
Snacks ___________________________

Friday

Breakfast ___________________________
Lunch ___________________________
Dinner ___________________________
Snacks ___________________________

Saturday

Breakfast ___________________________
Lunch ___________________________
Dinner ___________________________
Snacks ___________________________

Notes:

____
____
____
____
____

Weekly Meal Journal

week OF: ________________

Sunday

Breakfast ________________
Lunch ________________
Dinner ________________
Snacks ________________

Monday

Breakfast ________________
Lunch ________________
Dinner ________________
Snacks ________________

Tuesday

Breakfast ________________
Lunch ________________
Dinner ________________
Snacks ________________

Wednesday

Breakfast ________________
Lunch ________________
Dinner ________________
Snacks ________________

Thursday

Breakfast ________________
Lunch ________________
Dinner ________________
Snacks ________________

Friday

Breakfast ________________
Lunch ________________
Dinner ________________
Snacks ________________

Saturday

Breakfast ________________
Lunch ________________
Dinner ________________
Snacks ________________

Notes:

____
____
____
____

Weekly Meal Journal

week OF: _______________

Sunday

Breakfast _______________
Lunch _______________
Dinner _______________
Snacks _______________

Monday

Breakfast _______________
Lunch _______________
Dinner _______________
Snacks _______________

Tuesday

Breakfast _______________
Lunch _______________
Dinner _______________
Snacks _______________

Wednesday

Breakfast _______________
Lunch _______________
Dinner _______________
Snacks _______________

Thursday

Breakfast _______________
Lunch _______________
Dinner _______________
Snacks _______________

Friday

Breakfast _______________
Lunch _______________
Dinner _______________
Snacks _______________

Saturday

Breakfast _______________
Lunch _______________
Dinner _______________
Snacks _______________

Notes:

____
____
____
____

Weekly Meal Journal

week OF: ________________

Sunday

Breakfast ________________
Lunch ________________
Dinner ________________
Snacks ________________

Monday

Breakfast ________________
Lunch ________________
Dinner ________________
Snacks ________________

Tuesday

Breakfast ________________
Lunch ________________
Dinner ________________
Snacks ________________

Wednesday

Breakfast ________________
Lunch ________________
Dinner ________________
Snacks ________________

Thursday

Breakfast ________________
Lunch ________________
Dinner ________________
Snacks ________________

Friday

Breakfast ________________
Lunch ________________
Dinner ________________
Snacks ________________

Saturday

Breakfast ________________
Lunch ________________
Dinner ________________
Snacks ________________

Notes:

____

Weekly Meal Journal

week OF: _______________

Sunday

Breakfast ....
Lunch ....
Dinner ....
Snacks ....

Monday

Breakfast ....
Lunch ....
Dinner ....
Snacks ....

Tuesday

Breakfast ....
Lunch ....
Dinner ....
Snacks ....

Wednesday

Breakfast ....
Lunch ....
Dinner ....
Snacks ....

Thursday

Breakfast ....
Lunch ....
Dinner ....
Snacks ....

Friday

Breakfast ....
Lunch ....
Dinner ....
Snacks ....

Saturday

Breakfast ....
Lunch ....
Dinner ....
Snacks ....

Notes:

Weekly Meal Journal

week OF: _______________

Sunday

Breakfast...
Lunch..
Dinner...
Snacks..

Monday

Breakfast...
Lunch..
Dinner...
Snacks..

Tuesday

Breakfast...
Lunch..
Dinner...
Snacks..

Wednesday

Breakfast...
Lunch..
Dinner...
Snacks..

Thursday

Breakfast...
Lunch..
Dinner...
Snacks..

Friday

Breakfast...
Lunch..
Dinner...
Snacks..

Saturday

Breakfast...
Lunch..
Dinner...
Snacks..

Notes:

Weekly Meal Journal

week OF: _______________________

Sunday

Breakfast
Lunch
Dinner
Snacks

Monday

Breakfast
Lunch
Dinner
Snacks

Tuesday

Breakfast
Lunch
Dinner
Snacks

Wednesday

Breakfast
Lunch
Dinner
Snacks

Thursday

Breakfast
Lunch
Dinner
Snacks

Friday

Breakfast
Lunch
Dinner
Snacks

Saturday

Breakfast
Lunch
Dinner
Snacks

Notes:

Weekly Meal Journal

week OF: ________________

Sunday

Breakfast ....
Lunch ....
Dinner ....
Snacks ....

Monday

Breakfast ....
Lunch ....
Dinner ....
Snacks ....

Tuesday

Breakfast ....
Lunch ....
Dinner ....
Snacks ....

Wednesday

Breakfast ....
Lunch ....
Dinner ....
Snacks ....

Thursday

Breakfast ....
Lunch ....
Dinner ....
Snacks ....

Friday

Breakfast ....
Lunch ....
Dinner ....
Snacks ....

Saturday

Breakfast ....
Lunch ....
Dinner ....
Snacks ....

Notes:

Weekly Meal Journal

week OF: ________________________

Sunday

Breakfast ___________________________
Lunch ___________________________
Dinner ___________________________
Snacks ___________________________

Monday

Breakfast ___________________________
Lunch ___________________________
Dinner ___________________________
Snacks ___________________________

Tuesday

Breakfast ___________________________
Lunch ___________________________
Dinner ___________________________
Snacks ___________________________

Wednesday

Breakfast ___________________________
Lunch ___________________________
Dinner ___________________________
Snacks ___________________________

Thursday

Breakfast ___________________________
Lunch ___________________________
Dinner ___________________________
Snacks ___________________________

Friday

Breakfast ___________________________
Lunch ___________________________
Dinner ___________________________
Snacks ___________________________

Saturday

Breakfast ___________________________
Lunch ___________________________
Dinner ___________________________
Snacks ___________________________

Notes:

____

Weekly Meal Journal

week OF: ___________

Sunday

Breakfast ____________
Lunch ____________
Dinner ____________
Snacks ____________

Monday

Breakfast ____________
Lunch ____________
Dinner ____________
Snacks ____________

Tuesday

Breakfast ____________
Lunch ____________
Dinner ____________
Snacks ____________

Wednesday

Breakfast ____________
Lunch ____________
Dinner ____________
Snacks ____________

Thursday

Breakfast ____________
Lunch ____________
Dinner ____________
Snacks ____________

Friday

Breakfast ____________
Lunch ____________
Dinner ____________
Snacks ____________

Saturday

Breakfast ____________
Lunch ____________
Dinner ____________
Snacks ____________

Notes:

____
____
____
____

Weekly Meal Journal

week OF: _______________________

Sunday

Breakfast ___________________
Lunch ___________________
Dinner ___________________
Snacks ___________________

Monday

Breakfast ___________________
Lunch ___________________
Dinner ___________________
Snacks ___________________

Tuesday

Breakfast ___________________
Lunch ___________________
Dinner ___________________
Snacks ___________________

Wednesday

Breakfast ___________________
Lunch ___________________
Dinner ___________________
Snacks ___________________

Thursday

Breakfast ___________________
Lunch ___________________
Dinner ___________________
Snacks ___________________

Friday

Breakfast ___________________
Lunch ___________________
Dinner ___________________
Snacks ___________________

Saturday

Breakfast ___________________
Lunch ___________________
Dinner ___________________
Snacks ___________________

Notes:

____
____
____
____

Weekly Meal Journal

week OF: ___________

Sunday

Breakfast ___________
Lunch ___________
Dinner ___________
Snacks ___________

Monday

Breakfast ___________
Lunch ___________
Dinner ___________
Snacks ___________

Tuesday

Breakfast ___________
Lunch ___________
Dinner ___________
Snacks ___________

Wednesday

Breakfast ___________
Lunch ___________
Dinner ___________
Snacks ___________

Thursday

Breakfast ___________
Lunch ___________
Dinner ___________
Snacks ___________

Friday

Breakfast ___________
Lunch ___________
Dinner ___________
Snacks ___________

Saturday

Breakfast ___________
Lunch ___________
Dinner ___________
Snacks ___________

Notes:

____
____
____
____

Weekly Meal Journal

week OF: _______________

Sunday

Breakfast _______________
Lunch _______________
Dinner _______________
Snacks _______________

Monday

Breakfast _______________
Lunch _______________
Dinner _______________
Snacks _______________

Tuesday

Breakfast _______________
Lunch _______________
Dinner _______________
Snacks _______________

Wednesday

Breakfast _______________
Lunch _______________
Dinner _______________
Snacks _______________

Thursday

Breakfast _______________
Lunch _______________
Dinner _______________
Snacks _______________

Friday

Breakfast _______________
Lunch _______________
Dinner _______________
Snacks _______________

Saturday

Breakfast _______________
Lunch _______________
Dinner _______________
Snacks _______________

Notes:

____
____
____
____
____

Weekly Meal Journal

Sunday

Breakfast _______________
Lunch _______________
Dinner _______________
Snacks _______________

Monday

Breakfast _______________
Lunch _______________
Dinner _______________
Snacks _______________

Tuesday

Breakfast _______________
Lunch _______________
Dinner _______________
Snacks _______________

Wednesday

Breakfast _______________
Lunch _______________
Dinner _______________
Snacks _______________

Thursday

Breakfast _______________
Lunch _______________
Dinner _______________
Snacks _______________

Friday

Breakfast _______________
Lunch _______________
Dinner _______________
Snacks _______________

Saturday

Breakfast _______________
Lunch _______________
Dinner _______________
Snacks _______________

Notes:

____
____
____
____
____

Weekly Meal Journal

week OF: ___________

Sunday

Breakfast ___________
Lunch ___________
Dinner ___________
Snacks ___________

Monday

Breakfast ___________
Lunch ___________
Dinner ___________
Snacks ___________

Tuesday

Breakfast ___________
Lunch ___________
Dinner ___________
Snacks ___________

Wednesday

Breakfast ___________
Lunch ___________
Dinner ___________
Snacks ___________

Thursday

Breakfast ___________
Lunch ___________
Dinner ___________
Snacks ___________

Friday

Breakfast ___________
Lunch ___________
Dinner ___________
Snacks ___________

Saturday

Breakfast ___________
Lunch ___________
Dinner ___________
Snacks ___________

Notes:

____

Weekly Meal Journal

week OF:

Sunday

Breakfast
Lunch
Dinner
Snacks

Monday

Breakfast
Lunch
Dinner
Snacks

Tuesday

Breakfast
Lunch
Dinner
Snacks

Wednesday

Breakfast
Lunch
Dinner
Snacks

Thursday

Breakfast
Lunch
Dinner
Snacks

Friday

Breakfast
Lunch
Dinner
Snacks

Saturday

Breakfast
Lunch
Dinner
Snacks

Notes:

Weekly Meal Journal

week OF: _______________

Sunday

Breakfast ___________________
Lunch ___________________
Dinner ___________________
Snacks ___________________

Monday

Breakfast ___________________
Lunch ___________________
Dinner ___________________
Snacks ___________________

Tuesday

Breakfast ___________________
Lunch ___________________
Dinner ___________________
Snacks ___________________

Wednesday

Breakfast ___________________
Lunch ___________________
Dinner ___________________
Snacks ___________________

Thursday

Breakfast ___________________
Lunch ___________________
Dinner ___________________
Snacks ___________________

Friday

Breakfast ___________________
Lunch ___________________
Dinner ___________________
Snacks ___________________

Saturday

Breakfast ___________________
Lunch ___________________
Dinner ___________________
Snacks ___________________

Notes:

____
____
____
____